Dancing
in the
Sonshine

Restoration from the Wounds of Abuse

Second Edition

A Biblical Response to

Childhood Abuse, Domestic Violence, Sexual Assault

Kimberly Davidson

Dancing in the Sonshine: Restoration for the Wounds of Abuse Rev. **9.0**
Copyright © 2015; Revised: 2019 by Kimberly Davidson.
All rights reserved.

All Scripture quotations, unless otherwise indicated, are taken from the Holy Bible, New International Version®, NIV®. Copyright © 1973, 1978, 1984, 2011 by Biblica, Inc.™ Used by permission of Zondervan. All rights reserved worldwide. www.zondervan.com The "NIV" and "New International Version" are trademarks registered in the United States Patent and Trademark Office by Biblica, Inc.™

Scripture quotations marked (MSG) are from *THE MESSAGE*. Copyright © by Eugene H. Peterson 1993, 1994, 1995, 1996, 2000, 2001, 2002. Used by permission of NavPress Publishing Group.

Scripture quotations marked (NLT) are taken from the Holy Bible, New Living Translation, copyright © 1996, 2004, 2007 by Tyndale House Foundation. Used by permission of Tyndale House Publishers, Inc., Carol Stream, Illinois 60188. All rights reserved.

Scripture quotations marked (TLB) are taken from The Living Bible copyright © 1971. Used by permission of Tyndale House Publishers, Inc., Carol Stream, Illinois 60188. All rights reserved.

Scripture quotations marked (GW) are taken from GOD'S WORD®. Copyright ©1995 God's Word to the Nations. Used by permission of Baker Publishing Group. All rights reserved.

Scripture quotations marked (ISV) are taken from the Holy Bible: International Standard Version®. Copyright © 1996-2012 by The ISV Foundation. All Rights Reserved Internationally. Used by permission.

Unless otherwise designated, all Scripture quotations are taken from the New International Version (NIV) and the New Living Translation (NLT).

Cover Design by Mike Hodder
Interior Design by Kimberly Davidson

ISBN: 9781792933677

Contents

Stage One: Awareness & Education

1:	Hell on Earth	7
2:	Recognize and Respond to Abuse	26
3:	And Down and Down It Goes	43
4:	The Ways We Respond to Pain	55
5:	Is Your Love Tank Empty?	79

Stage Two: Mourning & Transition

6:	Healing from Loss of Love	96
7:	The Way of Transition	115

Stage Three: Resurrecting the True Self

8:	Hustling for Our Worthiness	133
9:	Sexual Shame Off You!	155

Stage Four: Transforming Beliefs

10:	The Power of Changed Beliefs	170
11:	Set Yourself Free with Forgiveness	186
12:	Change Your Mind and Memory—Change Your Reality	202

Stage Five: Reconnecting & Repair

13:	Things I Wish I'd Known About Love	223
14:	Receiving the Right Kind of Love	234
15:	Our Final Moment	248

APPENDICES

Appendix A: Feeling Wheel — 249

Appendix B: Deep Breathing — 251

Appendix C: Warning Signs of An Unhealthy and Abusive Relationship—Protecting Yourself — 253

Appendix D: Profile of an Abuser and Predator — 267

Appendix E: The Six R's to Authentic Change — 287

More Information—About Kimberly — 293

"My Notes" — 295

References — 297

Lord God, I pray You use the words in this book to penetrate and transform each reader's heart and mind, and clearly show her need for You Jesus, giving You all glory and honor. Amen.

Getting the Right Help

This study is not intended to take the place of medical or psychological care. For some of you, this study will be all you need. For others this may be one part of your overall healing plan. God's treatment on a spiritual level is critical to restoration yet is one component of a comprehensive care plan and does not come with a 100% healing guarantee. *Healing timelines and responses vary from person to person.*

Complex medical issues, trauma and *complicated grief* require more than the tools we explore in this book. In cases where there has been compounded trauma, it takes time to figure it all out. Consider seeking medical and therapeutic help. Licensed clinical counselors are trained to treat the difficulties associated with emotional pain.

If you are feeling depressed or extreme distress and/or are in therapy for a complex traumatic problem or feel you might have one, such as PTSD or an anxiety disorder, please don't do the suggested exercises unless a therapist clears you to do so. You may choose to use this material to understand yourself, and recognize why negative states of mind happen to you and millions of other people.

If you are in a group, some women who have a history of trauma can take on the emotions of the group and feel re-traumatized. Again, pray and decide what is the best course of action for you. It is also your responsibility to obtain professional resources in your community.

It's okay to not feel okay; there's no shame in seeking help.

**If you ever feel suicidal, seek help immediately.
Call 1-800-273-8255 or 911.**

IT IS TIME!

"Many of life's failures are people who did not realize how close to success they were when they gave up." –Thomas Edison

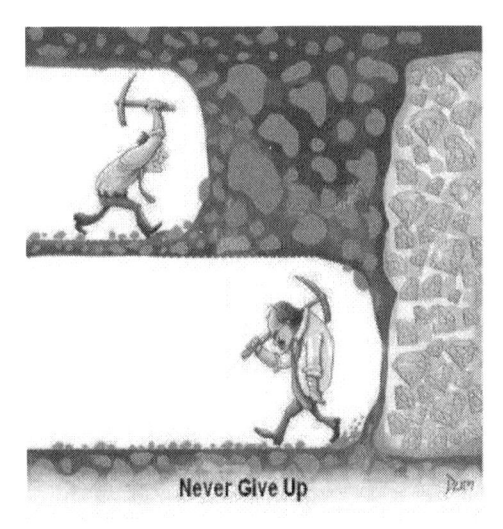

Often people think they are lost. They think that nothing in the world can help them. *And then God looks and says, "It is time."* And all at once everything looks different. Everything comes into a different light, and all at once you see that all is not lost, but won. Remember this, all is not lost in his eyes. The lowly shall be lifted up, the last shall be first."

— Ger Koopman

"Let today be the day you love yourself enough to no longer just dream of a better life; let it be the day you act upon it"
–Steve Maraboli

... Do not fear, my friend, Jesus Christ said, *"Let us go over to the other side (of the lake)" (Mark 4:35)*—not "let's go to the middle of the lake to be drowned." Get your hearts ready for an incredible boat ride with Jesus over to the other side of grief and sadness.

(See "Contents" for the road-map.)

1

HELL ON EARTH

There is a time to weep and a time to laugh, a time to mourn and a time to dance. – Ecclesiastes 3:4

Why is abuse such a widespread problem? Why are so many smart women caught in debilitating relationships? And why do some women allow themselves to be "reprogrammed" by an abuser?

Authorities claim today abuse and relational trauma is an epidemic. On a typical day, there are more than 20,000 phone calls placed to domestic violence hotlines nationwide.[1] How many more are suffering in silence?

There is definitely a spotlight on the subject, thanks to technology and the #MeToo movement. As the #MeToo movement continues, women are starting to see that people they know, love, and respect have also been victims of sexual assault. This has empowered more women to come forward and use their voices.

Were you aware that rape and abuse go back to biblical days?

Tamar took the nourishing dumplings she had prepared and brought them to her brother Amnon in his bedroom. But when she got ready to feed him, he grabbed her and said, "Come to bed with me, sister!

"No, brother!" she said, "Don't hurt me! This kind of thing isn't done in Israel! Don't do this terrible thing! Where could I ever show my face? And you—you'll be out on the street in disgrace. Oh, please! Speak to the king—he'll let you marry me."

But he wouldn't listen. Being much stronger than she, he raped her. No sooner had Amnon raped her than he hated her—an immense hatred. The hatred that he felt for her was greater than the love he'd had for her. "Get up," he said, "and get out!"

Oh no, brother, please! This is an even worse evil than what you just did to me!"

But he wouldn't listen to her. He called for his valet.

"Get rid of this woman. Get her out of my sight! And lock the door after her."

The valet threw her out and locked the door behind her.

She was wearing a long-sleeved gown. (That's how virgin princesses used to dress from early adolescence on.) Tamar poured ashes on her head, then she ripped the long-sleeved gown, held her head in her hands, and walked away, sobbing as she went.

Her brother Absalom said to her, "Has your brother Amnon had his way with you? Now, my dear sister, let's keep it quiet—a family matter. He is, after all, your brother. Don't take this so hard."

Tamar lived in her brother Absalom's home, bitter and desolate.

King David heard the whole story and was enraged, but he didn't discipline Amnon. David doted on him because he was his firstborn. Absalom quit speaking to Amnon—not a word, whether good or bad—because he hated him for violating his sister Tamar.

… Absalom prepared a banquet fit for a king. Then he instructed his servants, 'Look sharp, now. When Amnon is well into the sauce and feeling no pain, and I give the order 'Strike Amnon,' kill him.

… The king joined in, along with all the servants—loud weeping, many tears. David mourned the death of his son a long time" (2 Samuel 13: 1-22, 28, 37; MSG).

This tragic story highlights the problems and emotional cycle associated with sexual abuse and its aftermath. Not only does a man reap what he sows, but his children reap what he's sown also.

In that culture, the law mandated when a man raped an unmarried woman, he pays a dowry, marry, and never divorce her. Tamar was telling Amnon that by sending her away and not marrying her, he was destroying her future. Grieving, she tore her robe (a symbol of her virginity) and wept loudly. Historically, raped women have been considered "damaged goods."

Tamar's father, King David, was furious at Amnon, but did nothing; no scolding nor punishment. It's interesting that Absalom, another brother, at first discounted her emotions by saying, *"Be quiet now, my sister, he is your brother. Don't take this thing to heart" (13:20)*—yet, years later he took matters into his own hands.

King David neglected justice; Absalom implemented his own justice. He avenged Tamar by killing Amnon, resulting in many problems for himself.

History touches on the root of today's gender problem: the rule of man over the more vulnerable woman. One psychiatrist said, "Victims of abuse are taught that the strong can do as they please, without regard for the other person's soul." Rape was, and still is, strictly forbidden by God (Deuteronomy 22:28).

Anger, lust, and thirst for power motivated Amnon. And precious Tamar was left alone in a state of shock, weeping, mourning, and desolation. How sad that David didn't value and mourn his daughter's losses—her virginity, well-being, dignity and her future.

No one should experience what Tamar endured. What happened to her? Being raped by her brother and called "this woman" instead of her given name, and then being physically thrown out by a servant, no doubt, made her feel like damaged goods. A gigantic stronghold of shame, among other strong toxic emotions—perhaps even hate, consumed her.

The Bible says she lived in Absalom's house a ruined and desolate woman. *Ruined. Desolate.* Tamar lost hope. She never married or had children. In those days, a woman needed a man. Most likely, the symptoms stayed hidden or masked for years. Surely, she took this to her grave. Did she ever know God had a wonderful plan for her life?

The horrible secret things that happen in homes where we should have been safe, are not hidden from God, nor will they remain secret. First Corinthians 4:5 says, *"When the Lord comes, he will turn on the light so that everyone can see exactly what each one of us is really like, deep down in our hearts."*

† What about this story resonates with you most?

Abuse Today

Abuse is real, and sadly, far too common. Many therapists call it "relational trauma" because it's hell on earth and poison to the soul. The word "abuse" can be understood by breaking it down to *ab-use* or *ab(normal) use*. To abuse something means to use it for a reason other than it's intended purpose.

The story of Tamar begs us to reflect on rape myths of today, such as, *She wanted it. Guys can't control their urges. If she didn't scream or fight back, it wasn't rape. She didn't say no. Her clothes said she was willing.*

The voice of the enemy also fans the flames of despair: *Look at what you did! Can there be anything worse? There's no hope for you now. You're nothing—beyond redemption.*

The abuser may try to make the abuse look like an act of love, "I did it to keep you from ..." But those lies and blame-games and rationalizations are pure poison. Because God did not wire us, male and female, to be violated, *abuse is trauma.*

"Trauma" means that a person has *experienced a severe life event or situation that is emotionally painful and distressing, overwhelming the person's ability to cope, leaving her/him feeling powerless and out of control.*

Many of you can identify with Tamar. You can relate to her feelings of powerlessness; of silence. You know what it's like to be victimized in the place which should have been a place of safety and security. You know what it means to have those who should have protected you hand you over to save themselves. You know what the twisted despair feels like when an abusive person transfers their guilt and shame onto you. What you thought was true—counted on to be right—wasn't. It was outright deceit and lies. It was hard to tell because there was just enough truth to make everything seem right. *You're not alone!*

In America, we are saturated with untreated trauma and violence. Like cancer, it's deadly and can metastasize if left untreated. A high-level specialist in security issues, Gavin DeBecker, wrote,

> The energy of violence moves through our culture. Some experience it as a light but unpleasant breeze. Others are destroyed by it, as if by a hurricane. But nobody—nobody—is untouched. Violence is a part of America. It is around us and it is in us.[2]

Our restoration journey starts with *awareness* and *education*. Healing comes through understanding because once we can understand something, *we can control it* instead of allowing it to control us.

We'll begin by looking at the staggering statistics. *How many of these statistics reflect your story?*

- 1 in 3 females is sexually abused by the age of 18.
- 1 in 5 females have been assaulted.[3]
- A woman is beaten every 15 seconds in America.
- People who have experienced high rates of abuse/trauma have high rates of healthcare use. Women visit emergency rooms for injuries caused by intimate partners more often than for injuries from car accidents, robberies, and rape combined.
- A woman is killed every 2 hours by a stalking husband or boyfriend.[4]
- Rape is the most rapidly growing, yet underreported crime in America. 1 in 5 females are raped (compared to 1 in 71 males).
- 48% of all rapes involve a young female under the age of 18.[5]
- The Northwest states have the largest per-capita percentage of female victims who have suffered any form of sexual violence other than rape: *Oregon: estimated 56% of state's total female population; Washington: 53%.*[6] (2009 Gallup poll ranked Oregon as the state with the highest percentage of residents identifying with "No religion, Atheist, or Agnostic." Hmm … think there's a connection?)
- Women with a history of sexual violence report more severe symptoms of severe PTSD.
- There is a connection between online dating and sexual assault.[7]
- 25% to 33% of females experience *Domestic Violence* or *Intimate Partner Violence*; women ages 20 to 24 are at the greatest risk.[8]
- Nearly 70% of *all* reports of sexual assault occur to children ages 17 and younger.[9]
- Every 47 seconds a child is abused or neglected; every 5.5 hours a child is killed by abuse or neglect.[10]
- 90% of child sexual abuse victims know the offender; 70% are abused by a nuclear or extended family member.[11]
- *Over* 39 million adults in the US survived childhood sexual abuse.

Dancing in the Sonshine | 11

- 10 million children *witness* domestic abuse each year, which is now categorized as *emotional child abuse,* due to the adverse effects on the child. (Children literally take on the feelings of others due to the activation of *mirror neurons,* responding strongly to what they see).[12]
- In childhood sexual abuse, *total memory loss* happens in 19 to 39% of the victims.[13] (The younger the child at the time, and the closer the relationship to the abuser, the more likely she will not remember at all or not remember clearly.)
- Female child abuse survivors are more likely to be re-victimized.
- Childhood sexual abuse is a contributor in child prostitution.[14]
- Physical & sexual abuse are primary factors in adolescents running away and becoming homeless and contributes to youth suicide.[15]
- 52% of abused victims consider suicide; the abused make more (20-26%) suicide attempts.
- Within the military, sexual harassment/assault and rape have become significant. They call it: MST for *military sexual trauma.*
- Over 70% of people with disabilities say they've been abused.[16]
- Men too are victims and far less likely than women to report.

Unfortunately, far more souls suffer in silence. For every confirmed report, experts believe there's anywhere from 10 to 100 unreported cases stemming from feelings of shame, guilt and/or dependence on the perpetrator. Many view the justice system as closed to them, believing there is systematic bias and discrimination. I believe that if these statistics were cut in half, so would the prison population be cut in half.

Do What Your Gut Says

As a society we prefer to believe *"It can't happen here,"* maintaining our denial. The cost: damage inflicted on millions of people. Albert Einstein said, "The world is a dangerous place to live, not because of the people who are evil, but because of the people who don't do anything about it." It's critical to report a crime.

Research shows a woman's *intuitive sense* of whether her partner will be violent with her and/or her children is a substantially more accurate predictor of future violence than any other warning sign. The root of the word *intuition* means "to guard; to protect."

Listen to your gut! Experts say, when we are faced with a decision and there's not any reliable data, we should take our gut feelings seriously. They are often the first to tell us there's a problem with someone's behavior. However, we tend to override our intuition.

Not too long ago a young man approached me at a grocery store and asked if he could help put my groceries in my car. My gut said, *This is weird. I don't look helpless.* I answered, "No thank you."

One second later my mind switched, *He's probably some nice Christian guy wanting to help.* All I know is he was a stranger (as in "Stranger Danger").

† What is your biggest takeaway from this information?

To Become Like God

The main reason a woman becomes trapped in an abusive relationship is because a skilled offender has decided to target her. –Don Hennessy

It all started in the Garden of Eden when Satan (disguised as a serpent) got the first human beings, Adam and Eve, to question God's motives for giving a command to not eat the forbidden fruit hanging on the "tree of knowledge of good and evil" (Genesis 2:17). *He said to the woman, "Did God really say 'You must not eat from any tree in the garden'? (Genesis 3:1).*

The devil asked Eve to challenge the facts and the truth, to which she replied, *'We may eat fruit from the trees in the garden, but God did say, 'You must not eat fruit from the tree that is in the middle of the garden, and you must not touch it, or you will die' (Genesis 3:2-3).*

Then the serpent declared, *'You will not certainly die … For God knows that when you eat from it your eyes will be opened,* **and you will be like God,** *knowing good and evil' (Genesis 3:4-5).*

Dancing in the Sonshine | 13

I think it was the excitement of becoming like God overrode good judgment. Adam followed suit. The couple accepted without investigation what the serpent implied and proceeded to act upon it.

This is the truth: Adam and Eve lived in the *perfect* environment. They were already like God! *"God created man in his own image, in the image of God he created him; male and female* [Adam and Eve] *he created them ... When God created mankind, he made them* [Adam and Eve] *in the likeness of God" (Genesis 1:26-27; 51).*

By suggesting Eve eat the forbidden fruit, the devil's aim was to get both Adam and Eve to doubt who they were, and also agree with him in opposition to God, thereby, empowering him. These are the same words the devil today instills in an abuser's mind: *You have the right to be as powerful as God—and get your woman to focus on you only.* To this day, by agreeing with the devil's lies, an abuser is able to *"kill, steal, and destroy" (John 10:10).*

The Male Intimate Abuser

When I use the term "abuser" I'm speaking of a person who has *recurring problems with disrespecting, controlling, insulting, devaluing, or harming their partner, child, or another person.* Their real achievement is they've managed to adapt their tactics to fit their culture.

Abusers may look powerful and together on the surface, but on the inside they're often insecure, afraid, walled off by pain, grief, and fearful of losing control and being vulnerable.

Their childhood histories often include chaotic, neglectful, controlling or abusive families. Many experienced chaos or witnessed horrendous abuse in their own childhood and have developed distorted values. They're desperately attempting to purge their own pain. Savannah said, "My mother communicated only sarcastic remarks and put-downs. This is how she spoke and how she taught me to speak to my children and husband."

Humans always find ways to feel important, even grandiose. So, these wounded children often find it through being an adult perpetrator of violence. Psychotherapist Mike Lew explains:

He feels he must achieve power to avoid further victimization. In a world divided into victims and perpetrators, abuse can be interpreted as power. *The only way of masculinizing (empowering) himself is by turning someone else into a victim.* As terrible as it feels to be an abuser, *it feels like his only chance to leave the role of victim.* He never wants to play the victim again.[17]

If we dare to hold them accountable, we hold up a mirror to their own fears and fixed-mindedness. So, they react by abusing us instead of examining themselves. The victim becomes convinced that it is her behavior that triggers his abuse that she is deflected from examining his behavior. Proverbs 14: 22 states, *"Do not those who plot evil go astray? But those who plan what is good find love and faithfulness."*

Those who commit abuse are just as trapped in unhealthy beliefs and hurts as those they wound. Their dysfunctional thinking and behaviors only make sense to themselves.

Emotionally unstable people too have an innate need to be loved and feel secure, but sadly, little ability to nourish or nurture healthy relationships. They "strain and drain" and "engage and enrage."[18]

At the core of their evil and wrongdoing is the desire to be God, rather than serve and worship God. This is why they need to be reported, held accountable for their actions, helped by professionals, and possibly incarcerated for the safety of the families and community. Even though human behavior can be explained by what precedes it, it doesn't excuse it.

God is outraged by abuse because the human soul which He created, *in His image,* is dishonored and violated. Bondage is never the heart of God for His people. He wired us for loving relationships, to stay connected to others and Him. He created the pleasure centers of our brains to light up when we're in nurturing relationships. He calls each one of us to a life of freedom and personal transformation. *This is why abuse is so damaging—because a healthy connection has been broken.*

† You may be reading this and realizing, perhaps for the first time, that because of the abuse you've endured, you have become abusive. What do you believe God would say to you? (He gives you grace!)

"Empathy Erosion" – Turning People into Objects

The Director of the National Domestic Violence Intervention agency, Don Hennessey wrote, "I have been impressed at the sheer ability and ingenuity that these skilled and devious abusers have to gain access to a victim's mind, and their ability to avoid any unwelcome consequences of their abusive behavior."

How is it that some people can be capable of causing extreme hurt and torture to another person? One reason: "Empathy erosion."

Dr. Simon Baron-Cohen, a researcher and expert on the emotion of empathy, doesn't like the term "evil" and prefers to call human cruelty "empathy erosion."[19] *Empathy* essentially is when we comprehend and identify with what another person is thinking or feeling, and then respond to them with an appropriate emotion.

Dr. Baron-Cohen states "empathy erosion" comes as a result of fear, of beliefs we hold, and psychological characteristics. He emphasizes that when you treat someone like an object, their emotional empathy is turned off. "For them, self-focus is *all* that is available, as if a chip in their neural computer were missing."

The person who comes into contact with a person with empathy erosion is being on the receiving end of verbal assaults, physical attacks, or experiencing a lack of care or consideration.[20] There is a small percent of the population who have *zero empathy* because they have a personality disorder (narcissist, borderline, psychopath). Usually, beliefs drive cruel behavior with most of the unempathetic population. But their empathy circuitry may also be misfiring. To overcome, God and therapy is required.

† How does this make you feel about your abuser? Might you also recognize that you're not "crazy" as you've been led to believe?

The Future

I believe God is more interested in our future than our past; more concerned about what we can become than what we have been.

But—*your past is not your past if it's still infecting your present.* When the past demands our attention, it's best to respond. NYU neurologist Dr. Souhel Najjar regularly states, "You have to look backward to see the future."

No amount of stuffing, denial, or self-medicating will put an unhealed past away. I believe good counseling doesn't poke excessively into the past—only when the past is related to the present. Bringing up past events can help us see where our lives went out of control, and where we need the most work to ensure a healthy future. The past can't be undone and is part of who we are today. Yet, we can change our story's ending. First, we have to understand our story before we can change it.

Healing can only occur when our wounds are revealed.

Arlene Drake, a childhood abuse and trauma specialist wrote:

> Yes, you are a survivor, and there's much to be said for that. You made it through hell, and that took incredible resilience. Yet surviving with all the aftereffects of abuse isn't restoration. You deserve the true liberation that's earned by coming to terms with the pain of having been a victim, and doing the hard job of working through it, until you reach the freedom on the other side.[21]

I will be asking you to go to some scary places. *Please trust the process.* Remember, you can't patch a wound of the soul with a band-aid. Take away the main principles and ideas from the material. Don't get lost in the details. *God will enable you to understand and process the precise information He wants you to.* If at any time you start to feel overwhelmed or triggered, step away. Pray and apply the self-care deep breathing exercises in Appendix B.

Acknowledge your courage to take time out from your life to honor yourself by choosing to participate in this abuse restoration study. Be assured—*you're going to be okay.*

As they say, every cloud has a silver lining. Cowboy legend John Wayne once said, "Courage is being scared to death and saddling up anyway"—saddling up with Jesus! And someone else said, "There'd be no Savior if there wasn't a need for one."

Knowledge is Power

Throughout this book I reference brain science, called *neuroscience*. To heal from painful experiences, it's very helpful to know what happened on a biological (biochemical/brain) level, and where the abuse left imprints that have affected the way we experience life.

God has created our brains with the ability to recondition and rewire themselves on their own over time—*no matter our age!* This means the changes we make in our thoughts and behaviors can last as we create new brain structures and circuits. How? Knowledge.

Awareness and information are keys to transformation. It gives us the *power* to change—*if* we so desire. The Bible says, *"My people are destroyed from lack of knowledge" (Hosea 4:6); "You can't heal a wound by saying it's not there" (Jeremiah 6:14)*. Lack of knowledge is the reason we have conflict and get stuck. Knowledge is the investigation of the truth and often the truth hurts—but it also sets us free.

Knowledge is wonderful, but with it comes with responsibility. Knowledge—truth—alone doesn't counter the agony that is hidden in your heart or the decades of negativity playing in your head. To heal, we have to go through *a process*.

Let's look at this verse in its entirety. John 8:31-32 states,

> *Then Jesus turned to the Jews who had claimed to believe in him. "If you stick with this, living out what I tell you, you are my disciples for sure. Then you will experience for yourselves the truth, and the truth will free you" (MSG).*

What do you notice? There is a condition attached: *If you stick with this, living out what I tell you.* In other words, we have to live and follow the truth—God's Word, not merely stick it in that big encyclopedia in our skull …. Then we can be set free.

We begin to clearly see why we react the way we do and understand our responses to triggers and trauma. *[A "trigger" is when a file cabinet of memories is opened up, spilling out all the unpleasantries of those past events (my definition)].*

Counseling means I often don't tell women what they want to hear. Inevitably they put their "resistance" armor on. The purpose of bringing up experiences and feelings is not to bring back painful memories and relive the anguish, but to *get through to the other side*. It's not about reliving; just remembering. There's a saying "Feel it so you can heal it."

I recognize we all have life challenges, and some will be able to dedicate more time to this work than others. Obviously, those who make a commitment to do the work, change and heal faster. Yet, if you are one of the challenged, let me encourage you. A big of part change is *awareness* which can lead to daily progress and ultimately some life changes.

"I've Got You Sister!"

God's suffering servant Job anguished, *"I must express my anguish. My bitter soul must complain" (Job 7:11).* You will be encouraged throughout this book to talk about your losses. We are healed of grief only when we allow ourselves to express it—called "mourning." *Mourning* is the *outward* expression of grief. *I cry. I talk about what happened. I work through recovery exercises. I attend a healing Bible study.*

Real healing comes in the community of others as you face the darkness of what you don't understand with others who see and hear you; love and accept you; it's where we experience compassion and encouragement. Compassion literally means "to suffer with."

Think about this: How often do we cry out to God and ask, "Why don't *You* do something?" Too often we don't hear His response: *I am doing something—through the Church; through the people who belong to Me!* 1 Corinthians 12:7 says, *"A spiritual gift is given to each of us so we can help each other."* His power flows from human vessels—from your sisters in Christ.

God promises to *"comfort all who mourn and provide for those who grieve. He'll give them a crown of beauty instead of ashes, the oil of joy instead of mourning, and a garment of praise instead of a spirit of despair" (Isaiah 61:2).*

How might He do that? *"The God of all comfort, who comforts us in all our troubles, so that we can comfort those in any trouble with the comfort we ourselves have received from God" (2 Corinthians 1:3-4).*

"Comfort" in Greek means to encourage or please. Through others, God wants to come deeper and wrap you in His comfort. And we, the comforters, benefit too, *"Those who refresh others will themselves be refreshed" (Proverbs 11:25).* It begins with courageously asking for help.

Healing is a personal journey, no matter how minor it may appear. It must be respected. Feeling safe is key for everyone. When women start to share their feelings about pain in a group, it's very important to have a sense of safety. So, let's commit to be sensitive to each other's fluctuating emotions and share thoughtfully (avoid "oversharing," which means not revealing an inappropriate and/or shocking amount of detail about our personal life). Women connect through sharing weaknesses and vulnerabilities. It's important to commit to be a safe and supportive person; to be real versus right.

Younger women listen to the older women. Many of them have learned how to work with their emotions and deal with relationships more skillfully. They've experienced decades of navigating life's challenges and have wisdom to share. As Pastor Craig Groeschel said, "We're all terribly broken, yet brilliantly bright!"

Can you name a few people outside your group who can support you emotionally and spiritually through this process?

† What fears do you have about sharing your emotions and story?

Jesus Empathizes

We all know the Christmas story (see Luke 1). Mary, a virgin, bore our Savior Jesus Christ. Despite the stigma and the unanswered questions about the father, Joseph still married Mary. (Let's not forget an angel appeared to him in a dream and told him, *"Do not be afraid to take Mary home as your wife, because what is conceived in her is from the Holy Spirit."*)

Considered by some to be a "woman of ill repute," she endured the looks and thoughts of judgment and condemnation—that never diminished—from the people back home because she broke the law. They never knew the angel of the Lord had told Mary, *"You who are highly favored! The Lord is with you."* If they heard the story, it's doubtful they believed it.

The point is: Jesus was born out of wedlock—an illegitimate bastard—to this woman of so-called "ill repute." I believe His childhood experience gave Him a unique filter to understand and deal with victims. I know He has a deep heart for women who have been trampled by society. For decades I lived without a future and without hope— "a woman of ill repute" … until Jesus. He saved my life.

I stake my life on the power of the God of the Holy Bible to heal. One of His Hebrew names is Jehovah Rapha which means "The Lord that heals."

My role as a survivor and pastoral counselor is to teach, help, pray, and fight for you. Through this book, I give you everything I have (my gifts, heart, mind, passion, and training) because I want you to experience the miraculous just as I did.

The Bible, Our Foundation

One of Dorothy's classic lines in the *Wizard of Oz* is, "Toto, we're not in Kansas anymore." The Bible is the foundation of this study. For many of you, it may feel like you've left Kansas. I don't know your background or your understanding of the Bible. Give the Bible the benefit of the doubt; treat the text as reliable. My prayer is you embrace God's truths as you work through this study.

It is God's full revelation to us, telling us everything we need to know to live this life. When we read and meditate on the Word of God, we hear Him speak to us. It's that simple and that astounding.

The overall message is that Love (God) creates, heals, and renews; and frees believers from having to accept their "lot" in life. God wants a *relationship* with us, which is designed to lift us up and set us free, not fix and bind. God sent His Son Jesus to us, who said, *"The thief comes only to steal and kill and destroy; I have come that they may have life and have it to the full"* (John 10:10).

I know life's a big mess right now—and Jesus *loves* you. He wants a relationship with you. And yes, He *likes* you too! He wants to hang out with you, even when things aren't perfect in your life. Matthew 20:32 reads, *"Jesus stopped and called, "What do you want me to do for you?"* He's asking you the same thing. Be specific with your request.

There's nothing we can do, or fail to do, that can destroy our relationship with God (except to walk away from Him completely). *He can take who you are, no matter what you've done, and transform you into someone that no one else thought possible.* Before long people will notice a change in your personality.

* It wouldn't be unusual if you were a bit confused between who God is, who Jesus is, and who the Holy Spirit is. Please read this note (#22 in "References") if you are.[22]

† *When he had gone indoors, the blind men came to him* [God], *and he asked them, "Do you believe that I am able to do this?"*
   "Yes, Lord," they replied (Matthew 9:28).
   Do you believe, really believe, Jesus can help you heal? Explain.

"Pump You Up"—Or Not?

If you were a *Saturday Night Live* fan from the 1990's you no doubt remember, "Pumping it up with Hanz and Franz—the training program for the serious weight lifter." Most all of us, at one time or other, have attempted to "pump ourselves up," and not always with desired results. Listen to this diary entry:[23]

Dear Diary, I finally joined the local health club. I'm determined to drop 10 pounds and tone up. I want to look like I did 5-years ago. I made an appointment with a personal trainer named Antonio, a 26-year-old aerobics instructor and model for athletic clothing. I can't wait to begin!

MONDAY: *Tough to get out of bed at 5 A.M. but found it was well worth it when I arrived at the health club to find Antonio waiting for me. He is gorgeous! He showed me the machines. I enjoyed his aerobics class immensely. He's very inspiring! He encouraged me as I did sit-ups, although my gut was already aching from holding it in the whole time he was around. This is going to be a fantastic experience!*

TUESDAY: *Wearily, I drank a whole pot of coffee, but I finally made it out the door. Antonio made me lie on my back and push a heavy iron bar into the air then he put weights on it. Ugh! My legs were a little wobbly on the treadmill, but I made the full mile. His rewarding smile made it all worthwhile. I feel good!*

WEDNESDAY: *I dragged myself out of bed. The only way I could brush my teeth is by laying the toothbrush on the counter and moving my mouth back and forth over it. I think I have a hernia in both pectorals. Driving was okay as long as I didn't have to steer or stop. Antonio's voice is a little too perky for me this morning. He put me on the stair "monster." Why the heck would anyone invent a machine to simulate an activity rendered obsolete by elevators? I just tuned him out.*

THURSDAY: *The torture master was waiting for me. I couldn't help being a half hour late. It took me that long to tie my shoes. He told me to work out with dumbbells. I ran and hid in the restroom for rest of my hour.*

FRIDAY: *I cannot stand the sight of Antonio. If there was a part of my body I could move without unbearable pain, I'd hit him. He told me to work on my triceps. I don't have any triceps; they died! He sent me to the treadmill, which, as it got going faster and faster, flung me off. Humiliating!*

SATURDAY: *A day off—Yay!*

SUNDAY: *Church today; no gym—Yay! I considered dropping my membership until I got a glimpse of myself in the mirror coming out of the shower. Could it be? Is that a bicep? I think my hips look a little smaller? Are my eyes deceiving me? I tried on a pair of jeans I hadn't worn in quite a while and they fit perfectly! I can't wait to get back to the gym tomorrow!*

When the going gets tough, the tough get going—or do they? *Resistance* is a powerful human reaction to challenging work. The exercises in this book can change your life, but many of you will resist doing them or will walk away completely from this book or your group.

Disruption is the key. Breaking free and changing in a dramatic way, that is, *disrupting yourself,* takes effort. It sounds destructive, but in fact, it's a fulfilling process that has immense benefits. You can choose to raise your pain threshold—because then you grow. You can choose to believe: *I can do anything through Christ's strength* (Philippians 4:13). You can create a space in your heart for your grief work and still live your daily life. *Disruption = Breaking Free.*

Martin Luther's wife said, "I would never have understood the practice of the Christian life and work, if God had never bought afflictions (disruption) into my life." God promises to work our pain into a new exciting plan. *"See, I am doing a new thing!" (Isaiah 43:19),* He proclaimed.

My objective is to help you name and normalize what you haven't had a name for, or you've felt has been abnormal. If you've been abused, then you've been lied to, manipulated, intimidated, insulted and belittled.

There are two key reasons we need to do this work: One, we need to clean the "yuk" out. It's therapeutic and healing. Evidence shows that avoiding trauma-related thoughts and feelings contributes to general emotional distress, PTSD and depression. And two, when we are presented with new learning, the brain and mind are transformed; thereby, our lives are transformed. The very act of seeking help reflects you have the inner strength to do this!

But you can't do this alone. No one else but Jesus comes close to meeting our greatest needs and longing. He invites *you* to know Him and find healing and ultimate freedom.

If we truly want to see breakthroughs in difficult and seemingly impossible situations, and break satanic strongholds, then we must use the power that only comes from Him, otherwise the walls of adversity will remain standing. He is *the one* who does the real work in us and our circumstances; He's the force for transformation.

†††

I am honored to be your leader and counselor. In 2003 I had a deep calling to empower women to transformational change. It is a privilege and responsibility that I don't take lightly. I heard it said that many books are written with the author's blood. I've lived six decades. Anyone who has lived this long has experienced blood loss— numerous and assorted losses. I know about abuse.

I certainly don't have all the answers and am limited by my own experiences, perceptions and beliefs. Even when teachers do their best, the only way to be healed and blessed by God and the Word is through prayer and the inner teaching of the Holy Spirit. He is faithful to help us know truth from error.

I do have confidence in the job God has given me because He assures me in 2 Corinthians 2:9 that His power works through my weaknesses. How? He either gives me counsel to impart to you or He'll speak through another wise woman in the group who will give you exactly what you need to hear.

… Let us strip off every weight that slows us down, especially the sin that so easily trips us up. And let us run with endurance the race God has set before us"
(Hebrews 12:1, TLB)

2

RECOGNIZE AND RESPOND TO ABUSE

The severe scourging [*a whip or lash for the purpose of inflicting torture and punishment*], with its intense pain and appreciable blood lost, most probably left Jesus in a pre-shock state. Moreover, hematidrosis [*the excretion of blood in the sweat*] had rendered his skin particularly tender. The physical and mental, as well as the lack of food, water, and sleep, also contributed to his generally weakened state. Even before the actual crucifixion, Jesus's physical condition was critical.[24]

A team of medical and theological professionals just described the torturous event, called "crucifixion," that Jesus Christ endured prior to His death on the cross. The Romans trained men, called "lictors," to inflict torture, called "flogging." A whip was designed to rip into skin and turn muscle to pulp.

As if pain from intense physical torture weren't enough, Jesus also endured the emotional pain of cruel humiliation and shame. The soldiers spat on Him, mocked Him, beat Him, cursed His name.

The cross came after the flogging. The torment of the crucifixion was so extreme that a word was invented to describe it: *excruciating*. To ensure the greatest amount of humiliation, crucifixions were always done in front of a watching judgmental public.

Completely naked, Jesus became the object of vulgar remarks, which the Bible writers understandably chose to omit from the record.[25] This happened because of Jesus's enormous love and compassion for us. Second Corinthians 1:3 describes Him as compassionate and the God of all comfort. The literal meaning of *compassion* is "suffering with."

His death came slowly and painfully—from exposure, exhaustion, and finally suffocation. What is it that God would have us know in this drama and trauma of Jesus's abandonment, torture and pain? He would want us to know that He suffers and weeps with us with a broken heart. *"We don't have a priest who's out of touch with our reality. He's been through weakness and testing, experienced it all—all but the sin"* (Hebrews 4:15; MSG).

Through His earthly ministry, He displayed extraordinary perception and sensitivity to read a person's heart. *"For he knew what was in a man"* (John 2:25). And today, He is in tune to our feelings; to our disappointments, brokenness, fears, sorrows and hates.

Jesus is one of us. As a man, He agonized, wept, thirsted and knew loneliness. He needed the power of God's love—just as we do. He gets it. Jesus is no longer on earth living as the God-man. *Jesus is God* which means His spirit is everywhere and living in every one of His believers. If we truly want to change, then we need to understand it requires trusting Jesus. He is *the one* who does the real work in us; He's the force for transformation.

We are promised in 2 Peter 1:3, *"By his divine power, God has given us everything we need for living a godly life."* The words "has given" means it's already been done; past tense—"everything we need." This means we can live out Philippians 4:13, *"For I can do everything through Christ, who gives me strength."* Christ is sufficient enough for us; we no longer have to depend on our own self-sufficiency.

† Jesus said, "*Here on earth you will have many trials and sorrows. But take heart, because I have overcome the world (John 16:3).*

How does knowing Jesus has experienced tormenting abuse deepen your knowledge and relationship with Him?

Types of Abuse

O.J. Simpson was killing Nicole for years—she finally died on June 12th.
—prosecutor Scott Gordon

Abuse takes many forms. Each form leaves devastating aftereffects: anxiety; low confidence, self-image and self-worth; relationship issues and broken trust; powerlessness; and there are physical consequences. Keep in mind that each type of abuse overlaps with *emotional abuse, which by far causes the greatest harm.*

We are now going to go through the types of abuse so you can identify the ways you've been wounded, abused, or victimized. By acknowledging and understanding each kind of abuse, you can begin to normalize what you've experienced.

Recognize there is a misconception that *abuse* means physical violence. Many women think that if their partner doesn't hit or push them around, they're not being abused.

The definition of *Intimate Partner Violence/Domestic Abuse* is "actual or threatened physical, sexual, psychological or stalking violence by current or former intimate partners."

Also recognize that the confusing thing about abusive behavior, particularly if you grow up with it, is you may think it's pretty normal.

As you go through each type of abuse, underline or circle the ones you have experienced (if you don't mind writing in your book).

Emotional/Psychological Abuse

Emotional abuse or "emotional trauma," is any non-physical behavior intended to manipulate, coerce, intimidate, threaten, undermine, and confuse; anything that interferes with independence, and is aimed at discrediting and silencing. It is difficult to prove and is *often mistaken for normal marriage conflict*—but is the opposite of love. Think of the acronym TIME: **T**hreat, **I**ntimidation, **M**anipulation, **E**scalation

A *threat* is a statement of an *intention to do harm*—period. *Intimidations* contain words such as *if, or else, unless,* and are statements of conditions to be met in order to avert harm. For example, "I will burn your new leather coat *if* you don't have sex with me now." With threats no conditions are offered and they carry a more likelihood of a violent outcome.[26]

Intimidation aims to change the behavior or perception of others through abusive, deceptive, or underhanded tactics and behaviors.

Manipulations are statements used to influence an outcome without resorting to threat. Lying is common. One woman said, "I'm always disappointed when a liar's pants don't actually catch on fire."

Manipulators guilt-trip, belittle, give the silent treatment, and/or make dire predictions. They may appear to make amends (promises, gifts, expressions of affection; "I can't live without you")—yet, he has no interest making amends. He is far more interested in improving his image or undermining his woman's character. Parents do this to their children too.

Fear is the essence of TIME which is an abuser's main tactic. The tone of voice or the raising of a finger or hand can raise one's anxiety and fear level.

Guilt is a powerful manipulation. Once an abuser plants seeds of guilt, he doesn't need to physically prevent a person from certain actions, like leaving, because her own guilt will do this.

There is what I call *optimistic manipulation*. This is when the abuser uses something positive like romance to distract you from your feelings. For example, if he brings you flowers to stop your criticizing his bad behavior. Or he insults you in front of his friends and immediately follows up with a great compliment that takes your breath away. Then he gets *you* to doubt your perception about the situation, and he looks like the good guy.

Escalations are actions intended to cause fear, upset, or anxiety, such as showing up somewhere uninvited or sending something alarming or damaging. For example, when controlling his wife's behavior no longer works, the husband escalates by trying to do anything to keep his wife from changing their relationship, such as keeping her isolated.

Abusers use "emotional blackmail" tactics such as: ridicule, sulking, accusing, interrupting, refusing to respond, not listening, laughing at your grievance, changing the subject, provoking guilt, yelling, swearing, playing the victim, name calling, walking out, extortion (threatens to disclose damaging information about you), abandonment.

Other behaviors are: constant monitoring, stalking, harassing, bullying; threatening to hurt or kill family members, not allowing her to speak, withholding intimacy (*touch deprivation*), giving out the silent treatment, and using children as pawns to get what they want.

Deflecting blame is a common tactic to transfer responsibility of abusive behavior to the victim—*You made me do this*. The victim willingly accepts it—*It's all my fault.*

Crazy making and Gaslighting: "Crazy making" through power and control is one popular abuser tactic. Abusers "gaslight," a tactic in which a person in order to gain more power, twists the truth to make a person question her reality and sanity. They redefine truth and get her to question her memory of what actually happened. In time, she begins to question her own ability to remember and becomes more convinced the abuser is right. Her insecurity about herself and idealization of him offer the perfect opening for his manipulation and brainwashing tactics. She has no idea why this is happening.

("The Gaslight Effect" is now a national term, after the 1944 movie *Gaslight* with Ingrid Berman and Charles Boyer.)

This is emotional manipulation in which the gaslighter tries to convince her that she's misremembering, misunderstanding, or misinterpreting her own behavior or motivations, thus creating doubt in her mind, which leaves her feeling confused and vulnerable. He distorts reality and demands that she agree with his distorted view. He acts as though he's done nothing; instead she is labeled the unreasonable one for being upset.

Gaslighters pretend to be on your side but then sabotage you. They insist you go along with their point of view you know isn't true, but you convince yourself it is true in order to win that person's affection. They display "high-conflict" passive-aggressive behavior.

When we live in a world of confusion and start to question our perceptions and sanity—we become easier to manipulate. This is because deception causes crazy-making. You're not crazy—just on a crazy train.

Brainwasher is another word to describe emotional abusers. Researchers have drawn parallels between the tactics used in prisoner-of-war camps to brainwash and breakdown their prisoners, with the strategy's abusers use to control their partners, or anyone they consider their "property." They subtly take a victim's mind captive and the victim soon adopts their abuser's point of view and embraces their perspective. Some women come to believe violence is an expression of love.

Abusers are always in control. The victim is stripped of any sense of control over her fate, leaving her feeling helpless and hopeless. The cumulative effect of repeatedly being denied one's own desires, and the pressure to conform, causes severe emotional distress. She gives up and lives as a walking corpse without any sense of purpose.

Experts agree therapy cannot counteract the brainwashing if she remains in the relationship. That's why *bringing God in is critical.*

Digital or Cyber-abuse uses technology to control: excessive texting, sexting, cyber-exhibitionism; using the Internet to bully, harass, stalk, manipulate, or intimidate, spying on and monitoring victims through the use of tracking systems, abusing victims on social media sites, sharing intimate photos of the victim without their consent (called "revenge porn").

Social abuse: Using manipulation and control to *isolate* and keep a person away from all healthy connections such as family and friends; or preventing her from participating in work, school, church, or other independent activities. An abuser usually wants the person home where she can be watched and controlled; where she becomes more dependent upon him—in order to keep "the secret." What happens is: Reality and truth get distorted when we're isolated.

Financial/Economic: Using money or access to accounts to exert power and control; interferes with the ability to get or keep a job or go to school.

Abandonment/Neglect can cause the same emotional damage as the other types of abuse. Under the AHA definition, if a child is consistently ignored, rejected, isolated, verbally assaulted, terrorized, neglected, or exploited, they are being abused, such as being forced to watch the abuse of other family members or being caught in the middle of a parent's fight.[27]

The CDC estimates that 25% of the children in America have been neglected, which is when a parent or guardian fails to meet a child's basic physical needs.[28] This involves someone in a position of power and responsibility failing to act morally and legally; failing to provide the child or adolescent with adequate emotional support and a healthy sense of self.

Typically, emotionally neglectful parents don't usually have the same meanness that emotionally abusive parents do. They don't intend to hurt their children. They just never dole out words of affection or comfort, or hug and touch the child; or they make all the decisions for the child.

It can be very difficult to spot emotional abuse. Most women find many reasons for putting up with bad behavior—this man is your soul mate and father of your children; this is your parent who you depend on to meet your basic needs—but deep inside you know you are being treated wrong.

Verbal Abuse
Verbal abuse is typically chronic verbal interaction from a close relation like a partner, family member, or friend, that is unwanted and makes a person feel some kind of emotional harm.

"*The tongue also is a fire, a world of evil among the parts of the body … With the tongue we curse human beings, who have been made in God's likeness.*" *(James 3:6, 9)*. Proverbs 15:4 speaks about the destructive power of words as having *"the power of life and death"* and *"crushes the spirit."*

Negative remarks and memories are strongly encoded in the brain and are the most difficult memories to eradicate.[29] Just like toothpaste can't be put back into the tube, once hurtful words of death are out, they crush the spirit. This is because the brain cannot distinguish emotional pain from physical pain. Words *can* wound as much as sticks and stones.

Verbal abusers attack their victims in disturbing, degrading, and revolting ways; they interrogate, injure, criticize, insult, confuse, threaten, demean, and degrade, assaulting the person's dignity and humanity—yet they may be charming in public.

Lundy Bancroft, author of *Why Does He Do That?* wrote, "Each verbal battle with an abuser is a walk through a minefield."

Vicious attacks shame and make a person unable to think things through or see issues clearly. Insulting, harsh abusive words always leaves scars. For example, telling a child, *"I was pregnant with you when we got married, and your dad cried for days."*

Physical Abuse
Physical abuse is defined as nonaccidental physical acts such as hitting, shoving, biting, strangling, kicking, or using a weapon with the intent to cause fear or injury.

Would it surprise you to know that many abusers say they feel *entitled* to use physical force and violence?[30] According to experts, they often "look" for an excuse to abuse. Instead of, "What you did makes *me* mad," they think "*You* did this wrong thing, therefore, you must be punished." An eye for an eye (entitlement).

An abuser's chaotic and disorganized thinking tells him/her the consequences are tolerable and that there are no other alternatives, so violence is justified. To other abusers, alternatives to physical violence might be any one of these other kinds of abuse. Many perceive their actions as favorable, and they like getting the attention.[31]

Property: Destroying, hiding, or throwing out personal property; slamming doors. Hurting or threatening a family member or pet. (Behavioral specialists say if someone kills a pet, consider the person very dangerous.)

Self-inflicted physical abuse: Through self-injury such as suicide attempts or other kinds of self-harm, the abuser's intent is to cause their victim or so-called "loved one" to suffer.

Sexual Abuse (includes Rape and Sexual Assault)

Sexual abuse is exploiting another person through sexual contact or coerced non-consensual sexual contact, completed or not. The CDC (2013) uses the term *sexual violence:* an attempted or completed rape, unwanted sexual contact or harassment.

Sexual intimidation is a common feature. Every person has the right to say *no* at any point in a relational encounter. When a person doesn't take no for an answer, they are guilty of sexual abuse.

Sexual abuse includes both touching and non-touching offenses: forcing the victim to touch the abuser's sexual parts, affairs, sexual jokes, pornography, exhibitionism, penetration with an object or animal; insisting the person dress erotically, prostitution. It also includes restricting access to birth control or condoms (called "contraceptive abuse"), non-disclosure of STD/HIV status, forcing or terminating a pregnancy.[32]

Some husbands force their wives to have sex which is rape. "There's a wolf in your bed" as they say. The woman's sexuality, integrity and rights are ignored. The bed is the battle ground where he feels he must have control. His rights and beliefs take precedence over hers. In time she accepts his interpretation of conjugal rights.

Deanna's fiancé continually demanded offensive sexual acts, which Deanna felt were disrespectful. He used pornography as an instructional tool to normalize the violations and teach her how to perform. At first, she pushed back, but his clever brainwashing maneuvers slowly demeaned her dignity and she gave in repeatedly.

A spouse who repeatedly engages in other sexual entities like strip clubs, prostitutes or pornography is a *sexual addict/sexual betrayer.*

The dire consequences: Sexual abuse forges a strong connection between sex and shame. There's no un-doing what she's been forced to do. Moving forward, it becomes hard to separate love from sex. She will often gravitate toward emotionally and abusive unavailable men because they are sickeningly familiar to her. Yet she most likely will not be able to enjoy the pleasure of sex due to the devastation of trust, and fear and anxiety. Pleasure and memories of being violated don't go together.

Many feel a hatred, disgust, or revulsion for their bodies, often accompanied by a desire to be cut-off from bodily and sexual experiences. Some women purposefully make themselves unattractive, usually because of their mistaken belief that rape and incest are brought on by physical beauty or provocative clothing. They think, *I don't want to feel or look like a sexual object for men's gratification.* This is a myth because power and control—not sex, is the abuser's motive.

The Bible makes a strong differentiation between sex that enriches the human spirit and that which degrades it. For it to be a blessing between two people it means that both people are fully consenting, and that it takes place in a context of respect, choice, and regard for each other's well-being.

Sex is God's most intimate and powerful bonding activity (Matthew 19:6), therefore, must be used reverently and with caution. This is why sexual assault causes damage far beyond anything else. First Corinthians 6:19-20 says, *"... your body is a temple of the Holy Spirit within you, whom you have from God."* (See also: *Psalm 11:5; Proverbs 1:15-19.*)

Sexual violation can be the worst life crisis a person ever faces because sexuality is so sacred. It is a heavy burden and so stigmatizing that many women do not report it. It's been said that *10 people are affected by one person's sexual abuse.*

Sex Trafficking/Prostitution: a person is used for sexual exploitation; sex is exchanged for money and amenities. It's also called "paid rape." Victims are sexually exploited in extreme ways and repeatedly abused. Commonly, the person is deceived, coerced or forced into sex trafficking through many means, such as the promise of a better life.

Spiritual Abuse

Spiritual abuse is any kind of deception and manipulation that overloads people with spiritual weights, thereby, damaging the person's relationship with God. When God, the Bible, and/or faith is used to distort, weaken, feed people lies and take away their choices, or destroy a person's sense of self, spiritual abuse is present.

Many people quote the Bible, but not everybody uses it for good. Cults and atheists quote it. The devil himself quoted Scripture to Jesus. Some use it to corrupt the truth; others as a weapon.

Spiritual abuse is a real phenomenon that happens in the Church. A spiritual abuser may or may not be a religious leader. Their underlying motivation is not spiritual enlightenment but *spiritual enslavement*. Any kind of *cult-like ritual abuse* falls under spiritual abuse.

1—Abuse occurs when a *person in a position of spiritual authority*, like a minister, misuses their authority to control, degrade, shame, coerce, or manipulate for *seemingly God's purposes*, which are just their own.

The Bible says they *"masquerade as servants of righteousness"* (2 Cor. 11:15) and *"their end will be what their actions deserve."* Someone said, "The only thing worse than a wolf in sheep's clothing is a wolf in a shepherd's robe." Abuse can also include clergy who, for example, tell a rape victim that she was the one who provoked the attack. Clergy can *unintentionally* emotionally rape their own members.

2—The second type of spiritual abuser may be a *non-clergy person*. Raichel's husband disallows her attending church services, questions her beliefs, misuses and quotes verses out of context to manipulate her, and has made false accusations to the pastor about her.

3—Then there's *legalism,* which may or may not be spiritual abuse. (It depends upon the situation.) Legalism, in a nutshell, is when people reduce Christianity to a set of rules (which makes Jesus mad). There's no love; only judgment. Legalists tend to throw a bunch of do's and don'ts based scriptures at you to show you just how sinful you are. They are what Jesus called *hypocrites*.

Legalism goes against Galatians 5:1 and John 3:16. John 3:17 tells us that Jesus came into our world to save us, not condemn us.

The Physical Aftereffects

Our bodies hear everything that our minds say. *Abuse is extreme stress (trauma) to the body.* When our stress response is stuck in overactivation it can cause a big health hit such as: chronic anxiety; sleep problems; brain fog and distorted cognitive function; digestive problems; sugar, fat, and salt cravings; hormonal problems; metabolic syndrome; high blood pressure; internal inflammation; immune system problems and auto immune diseases.

Our emotional biography becomes our physical biology. Could you ever *imagine* there could be a physiological connection between what happened when you were a kid and your body breaking down decades' years later? Together they write much of the script for how we live our lives out.

Research repeatedly confirms that the human body believes everything the mind says. The body remembers every adverse experience—going all the way back to childhood—which is why so many of us today are struggling with illnesses and disease.

It's a fact: *Healing is more difficult if we do not recognize that our past plays a strong hand in our adult health problems to day*—unless a force—God—enters our lives and frees us from our personal prisons.

In addition, when you're under chronic stress your brain is geared to go for sugar, fat, and salt foods by releasing a flood of feel-good nervous system chemicals (*serotonin* and *dopamine*) that calm your nervous system. This is why we call them "comfort-foods." But this comfort comes at a price. We become addicted to them, which typically causes us to pack on belly VAT fat (*Visceral Abdominal Fat*), a type of hidden fat that produces inflammatory *cytokines* that wreak havoc on our entire body.[33]

We're beginning to unpack the truth. The more you can see truth, the more you will feel in control of your life. To name the types of abuse you've experienced is to admit the truth; express the unspeakable; acknowledge the losses, thereby enabling the healing process to move forward.

† How does this list speak directly to a need or trial in your life?

If you are in a class do the "Types of Abuse" exercise now.

Betrayal Bonds (Stockholm Syndrome)

> *Gary had done it. He had taken possession of my mind, body, and soul. Now, without any resistance on my part, he could command me to do every perverted, unspeakable act his twisted mind could dream up. … Every night when he came back and untied me, when he took off the gag and blindfold, and gave me a hamburger, I felt immensely grateful. Even though Gary was the person locking me in the lion's den, his presence was the only thing that made me feel safe and provided relief. In my brainwashed and terrified state, I felt it was my duty to protect my master.* –Michelle Stevens, speaking of her sex trafficker father

How could someone feel that being beaten doesn't justify leaving? Why does a woman stay married to a power and control nut? Why does she minimize his behavior? Why do many women ignore their intuition to leave an abusive relationship? Ever think, "How could I be so stupid?" That's the question we often ask ourselves at the end of an abusive relationship. Actually, we really weren't so stupid at all. Most people don't understand the complexities of abuse.

One chief reason they stay is *the inability to recognize that abuse is killing them.* For example, the abuser might scold you for hours about your bad behavior. Then, once you're in tears he'll apologize profusely, "Please forgive me. I didn't mean it. I just can't stand the thought that I might lose you!" He might use gifts, sex, or other intimacies to restore your former closeness—a response you embrace with relief. *He isn't such a bad guy after all. He's pretty terrific.* In the abuse cycle this is called the "honeymoon phase."

The more upsetting the bad behavior is, the more welcome his good behavior seems to erase it and return you to the former "magical" days. *We tend to hold on to the good memories and toss out the bad.* Harvard researchers found that if things aren't so great, human beings will deceive themselves to make things look rosier. We deal with reality by unconsciously distorting the bad. We turn it around to, "It's not him, it's me," "He feels so bad."

Those distortions become our core beliefs which serve as protection by insulating us from harm. Distortions tend to stave off depression and helplessness—automatically and outside of our awareness.[34]

Eleven-year-old Jaycee Lee Dugard was abducted from a school bus stop (1991). She went missing for over 18 years. Jaycee had two daughters by her abductor. Most people wonder why she didn't run away when she had the opportunity. The answer: she couldn't—not without help.

Psychologists have a term to explain this phenomenon: *Stockholm syndrome*. Other terms are "betrayal bonds," "trauma bonding," or "loyalty bonds." Exploitive relationships create "betrayal bonds" where people stay involved with people who betray them. Partners cannot leave one another when they clearly know the destructive risks. It is a painful situation for a person to depend on a protector who is at the same time the harmer. If she rejects the abuser, she loses her protector.

Betrayal bonds enable us to understand why a person doesn't leave or report their abuser. If someone holds your self-worth and life in their hands, they are a very powerful person to you. Pleasing this person becomes critical. Most of the time, she believes the abuser is protecting her instead of harming and dominating her. She can be so hungry for attention and love, her wounds so great, she doesn't see that the abuser has taken hold of her mind (brainwashing). She adopts his point of view because she believes she needs him to feel better about herself. She buys into his opinion of her as incompetent, ugly ... *[you*

Dancing in the Sonshine | 39

name it]. In a perverse way, she believes the abuser is helping, not hurting her. Often, the more severe and dangerous the abuse, the stronger the loyalty bond is because she idealizes him and is desperate for his approval.

These bonds are able to form because human beings have a biological need to form attachments with others. And if I'm convinced that I'm not good enough, I'll have a tough time accepting someone into my life who thinks I am. *Psychological domination* is the name of the game, primarily through threats and fear. *Control* creates fear, and fear deepens the bond. Due to the absence of any other points of view, the victim comes to see the world through the eyes of her abuser. If she does see the light, the thought of confronting or leaving him can feel too threatening to consider.

Then there's *bonding by terror*. Fear can actually immobilize and deepen attachments. The more frightened she is, the more she's tempted to cling to the relationship. In some cases, fear intensifies attraction and arousal, adding intensity and obsession.

History is full of examples of loyalty bonding. In the Bible, the Israelites showed signs of being trauma-bonded to their oppressors the Egyptians. When they were freed and led by Moses into the desert, they wanted to go back to Egypt (Exodus 16:2-4). Nine hundred people followed cult leader Reverend Jim Jones to their deaths. They were victims of violence, sadism, sexual exploitation, and murder—yet they followed.

Margie left her abusive husband multiple times. She recalls, "When I left, all I could feel was depression, sorrow, anger, numbness … even boredom. I'd have these terrifying nightmares and felt helpless. I figured I was so unhappy and having nightmares and flashbacks was because deep inside I missed my man. I didn't feel this way when I was with him, so I went back."

Many women are brainwashed and traumatized into believing that each horrible incident will be the last. (I recommend the book *The Betrayal Bond* by Dr. Patrick J. Carnes.)

There is another explanation: *addiction*—to either the abusive act, such as beatings or rape, or to the powerful feeling of overwhelming relief when the incident ends. In other words, the abuser holds the key to her feeling of well-being. In either case, powerful hormones are released in the brain which can make these actions addictive.

Some victims don't trauma bond. But they live in immense fear and don't feel they have access to resources to get out and stay out. They feel they're stuck and can't leave for reasons such as economic security, the children, or fear of abandonment and humiliation, for example. Betrayal bonding is not consciously chosen.

Learn to recognize any patterns of betrayal bonding in your life. Pray for wisdom.

† Many abused women struggle with a perceived change in their personalities. They fear they have changed into someone who is— whatever the abuser has repeatedly told them. How do you relate?

It Wasn't Your Fault ... and Never Was

Are you one of those women who believe that when bad things happen its verification that you're not worthy to be loved, respected, blessed, happy, peaceful or (fill in the blank)?

We need to get this: *Skilled offenders are the ultimate con men. We are not naïve or stupid for falling for their tactics.*

For abusers, attaining power *over* others is intoxicating. They are pros at poisoning our idea of who we are and destroying our thought life. *Abuse* is all about taking from others the good things God intended—namely their life, freedom and dignity.

When anyone who is in a position of greater power—strength, authority, or experience—violates a person's rights as a human being in any way, the behavior is abusive.

Abuse is a problem that lies with the abuser—not you. There is something terribly wrong with him or her. You never deserved it. You weren't stupid; you were innocent. The abuse wasn't your fault. You were a victim: Your weaknesses were exploited; you are normal; you are okay. There is much more to who you are than the abuse you've suffered!

If you are presently experiencing abuse, the problem will continue no matter what *you* try to change about yourself, your partner, or your relationship (marriage counseling rarely works). This is because the problem is the other person's abusive behavior—his need to control the relationship. Only he can choose to stop being abusive. This applies to any person in our life.

Often, we become the abuser in order to protect ourselves. Too often all this does is empower the abuser to do more harm.[35] Begin by trusting God. Start by letting God love you through this process. *You can trust Him.* He'll never force Himself on you. Evil forces itself—not Love. It's the road to restoration.

† † †

These few chapters may be particularly rough for you. But now that you know the worst, you are free to see beyond it. Being abused or assaulted is *not your fault;* nor is it God's fault. There are some things God has chosen not to reveal because we just can't understand His view—the supernatural view. *"The secret things belong to the LORD"* (Deuteronomy 29:29).

Pastor Matt wrote, "Will there still be questions without answers? Yes. But I don't think answers are what we are looking for anyway. I think we're looking for grace—enough so that we can manage the pain. And answers are not grace; they're just information."[36]

We need to remember that God *is* Love and Goodness. His ways are unpredictable yet trustworthy. Our job is to *trust*. God does not represent evil. *Evil is the absence of God; the absence of truth.*

3

AND DOWN AND DOWN IT GOES

If a father beats up his son, is that abuse? What if two siblings around the same age beat each other up, is that abuse? In the first case, it's abuse; in the second, it's fighting and cruel behavior, but not likely abuse. This is because there are two kinds of power.

The first one is "Power Over." For abuse to occur, it must *come from a place of higher power to a place of lesser power; there is a power differential.* People in low power positions cannot abuse people in high power positions. The father is in a power over position. Abusers *need* to have Power Over a person to feel complete. They use two of the most powerful human emotions—*love and fear,* to create an unequal power dominant relationship.

In chapter 1 we met Tamar's father, David, the one who did nothing about his daughter's rape. A story in 2 Samuel 11 may shed some light on his behavior and character.

Picture it: From his balcony, David sees a beautiful woman, Bathsheba, bathing. At that moment he "wanted" her. Verse 4 says, *"David sent messengers and took her."* Then he had his way with her. What he didn't plan on was a pregnant Bathsheba. So, to cover up his sin he had her husband murdered (so he wouldn't figure out he wasn't the father, since he was out fighting).

This is an example of "power over." He was king and she was his subject. Some call it "power rape." Eventually he recognized his sin and was remorseful (see Psalm 51).

The second kind of power is "Personal Power" which Jesus modeled. Personal Power shows itself as mutual respect and equality; it is attaining power *with* people. I am more interested in the person herself, than I am in controlling her. *Personal Power is "empowering."*

This reminds me of the popular Spider Man phrase, "With great power comes great responsibility."

Abuse is all about *power and control*. For these people, being in control is their only motivation. It's about taking away and making other people's choices for them; putting the victim in degrading and inhuman positions. What we don't realize is we come to feel safe because the other person does all the thinking for us; that's control.

This is not God's plan. He dislikes it when His people's freedom is stolen from them. His cry has always been, *"Let my people go" (Exodus 5:1)*. Our freedom comes from taking responsibility for ourselves; bondage comes from giving it away.

To be empowered is to be given back personal power and authority. It means we can hope and believe change is possible. We learn there are new and better ways to deal with these kinds of situations. *My objective for you as you go through this book is to be empowered, maybe for the very first time.*

† Describe how you feel right now. For example, hopeful, scared, empowered, or other.

Childhood Abuse and Adult Problems

The one I trusted for everything had let me down, so I decided I wouldn't trust anyone. Instead, I'd resist authority and never allow anyone close enough to hurt me like my father did. I was angry and resentful. Although I did later find the Lord, the pain and memory of that time in my life clung to me like a vine to a tree. I couldn't shake the pain or anger. I was a member of the "walking wounded." In some ways, I still am. People say to me, "Get over it," and you do to a certain degree. However, you never really get over it because Satan has a way of constantly reminding you of your weakness. He hits you where it hurts.

–Reverend H. B. London, Jr.

For centuries, children have been abused in their homes, and in most cases, it's well hidden.[37] This study isn't intended to focus on your childhood experiences, but rather your current experiences. You may be thinking, "Good, whether or not I was abused as a child doesn't change today's reality." You are somewhat correct.

What we need to realize is if we do have a history of abuse, abandonment, neglect and/or violence, this can lead to adverse results in adulthood because victimized children experience a corrupted childhood and damaged beliefs. They lose every child's right to experience a normal loving, protective, and nurturing childhood.

If you are a victim of childhood abuse, I want to give you a brief understanding of my perspective of why you feel the way you do and do the things you do in your life today. This can clarify many of our problems.

Before moving forward let me say that sometimes we resist looking at our childhoods because we're afraid we're dishonoring our parents. The search for truth—along with God—never requires we dishonor those who raised us. We must decide to become fearless in our search for the truth. The truth hurts but it also sets us free.

The Wounded Child

I grew up in a home where some painful things happened that no one talked about. Like a scene from The Wizard of Oz, my home was filled with flying monkeys. No one wanted to talk about them, or even acknowledge the monkeys existed.
–Dr. Sheri Keffer

Our family is the "deck of cards" God handed us, giving us virtually no say whatsoever. You may relate completely to the flying monkeys analogy Dr. Sheri used. Our parents didn't have a clue what they were signing up for when they brought us into this world or adopted us. Our parents, too, have to deal with their own history that was not of their choosing.

Parents (caregivers) have the most influence in building and shaping a child's brain. Think of a baby's new brain as a computer coming off an assembly line. It's waiting to download its new operational system. It will carry that initial programming it receives for life.

Wounded children typically *learn a distorted way of relating to others, and life in general.* They don't have the tools to handle rejection. Once beliefs have been damaged, they wander through life trying on and testing different masks to see what fits. It's not unusual for a victim to let herself to be revictimized in order to be close to *someone*. Sometimes, she may feel the only person she can get close to is the one who is abusing her, and/or the only possible intimacy is sexual.

One adolescent woman allowed her counselor to have sex with her. In her mind it was okay because he didn't beat, berate, or yell at her like her dad. The counselor's abuse felt like a caring, tender act. (He broke ethical boundaries.) This is an example of *learning a distorted way of relating to others.*

Abused children rarely recognize the problem is *not in themselves,* but instead in their chaotic upbringing. The parents' rights took precedence over the rights of the child. They remain trapped in a distorted self-image, carrying the weight of blame, anger, rage, and shame into adolescence and adulthood. It is in adulthood that they often suffer the most. The impact hits them as they search for genuine love, sexual intimacy, and commitment.

Today and Yesterday

Justine has no problems getting boyfriends. Her problem is keeping them. Now 25-years-old, she picks men with an edge who are emotionally unavailable. In every relationship she becomes clingy and her boyfriend eventually breaks up with her. Then she gets hysterical—she falls to the floor, puts her arms around his legs, pleading with him not to leave her.

Why such an aversive reaction?

With professional help, Justine eventually traced back the reason. She recalled one evening, when she was 6-years old, there was a dreadful thunder and lightning storm which terrified her. She called for her parents, but they didn't hear her because they were yelling and screaming at each other.

That stormy night Justine believed she was in danger. Her parents didn't come when she cried for them which gave her a feeling she'd been abandoned. In fact, their incessant fighting, gave her a recurring feeling that they weren't available when she really needed them.

This 6-year-old memory which was stored in her unconscious mind, became stimulated whenever a boyfriend broke up with her. At that point, she'd no longer function as a mature 25-year-old, but instead as a frightened little girl left alone in the dark.

Justine's therapist helped her make the connection between the storm, the fighting and a breakup. She unconsciously experiences breakups as "being in danger."

Negative reactions and behaviors in the present can be tracked directly back to earlier memories. They are called "unprocessed"—meaning they are stored in the brain in a way that still holds the emotions, physical sensations and beliefs that were experienced earlier in life. Identifying the memory connection is a first step towards healing.

Trauma and Memory Wars

If a client tells a therapist they have no recollection of whole pieces of their childhood, the therapist is immediately alerted to the possibility of some sort of abuse. A heavily debated topic in the field of trauma psychology is whether memories of childhood abuse can be lost and then later recovered, called *traumatic amnesia*. Studies suggest there are several factors associated with traumatic amnesia: age at time of abuse, severity and chronicity of abuse experiences, and lack of support at time of abuse.

It's widely accepted in both the clinical and scientific communities that experiences of childhood abuse and neglect are generally well-remembered. Among a small sub-group of individuals exposed to trauma, memories of abuse can be forgotten and later recovered.

"Forgetting the event," it is argued, can be explained by the failure of the young child to understand the nature of the abusive situation at the time. Or, they may have not been perceived the event as abuse at the time. The *betrayal trauma theory* proposes that when a child is traumatized by a close family member or caregiver, the child may be motivated to forget the trauma experience out of dependence upon and love for the abuser.[38]

Dr. Harriet Lerner, author of *The Dance of Connection*, wrote, "Children know at a deep, automatic level what they are not supposed to say or tell or even remember. Their utter emotional and economic dependency necessitates a fierce, unconscious loyalty to unspoken family rules."

I don't remember much under the age of seven, so I did some research. Research repeatedly states that young children tend to forget events more rapidly than adults because they lack the strong neural processes required to bring together all the pieces of information that go into a complex autobiographical memory.

It is about age seven when our earliest memories begin to fade, known as *childhood amnesia*. Therefore, if we cannot remember anything under 7-years-old, we can't automatically assume we were abused or traumatized. *False memories* also exist. Thus, some recovered memories may be accurate and true, while other recovered memories may contain errors or be false.[39]

† What about this resonates with you most?

Down It Goes

> *You [God] show unfailing love to thousands, but you also bring the consequences of one generation's sin upon the next.* –Jeremiah, speaking in Jeremiah 32:18

Every experience we've had in our lives has become a building block in our inner world, governing our reactions to everything and every person we encounter. When we *learn* something, the experience is physically stored within networks of brain cells called *neurons,* which form our unconscious mind—determining how our brain interprets the world around us, and how we feel from moment to moment which determines how we behave.

Our brains have been designed to mimic the emotional expression of others.[40] We learn thinking patterns and behaviors from our families. Called "the chameleon effect," we instinctively imitate others and mirror what we've observed, like exerting force as a means of maintaining control or venting frustration (anti-social behavior).[41] We don't know we're mimicking others.

Because of the "chameleon effect," children raised in abusive and violent homes are at a higher risk of becoming adult batterers. 85% of men who batter their wives, and 30% of their victims, grew up in violent homes.[42] Without intervention, generational abuse becomes part of a family's culture, mindset and identity.

Another factor is that our culture focuses on images of negative, violent, and high-conflict behavior. The media is teaching new generations that this is normal relationship behavior. What may be entertainment for adults is social training for kids.

It's been said, "Abusers are made, not born." Yet, there are *many* men (and women) who were abused as children and *don't* abuse their children and/or partners. *Although the majority of victims do not become perpetrators, clearly there is a minority who do*[43]—as high as 40%.[44] Figuring out why one kid in an abusive family turns into a perpetrator and the other into a good guy, is a coin toss.

† In what ways do you believe your childhood abuse continues to affect your adult life? (For example, do you go to great lengths to attain affirmation you desperately crave, but never seem to get? Are you an approval addict, overly compliant—a condition of "good-girl syndrome"?)

Changing Our Past

We shouldn't spend all our energy blaming our parents and environments for what we didn't get. This only keeps us stuck in a victim mentality and defocuses us from transformation and taking personal responsibility. Growth isn't about focusing on someone else's lesson; it's about focusing on our own. –Kimberly

There is no such thing as a perfect family where people don't get hurt. I believe in most cases that our parents parented us the best they could, given the emotional and physical resources they had, considering they were impaired from knowing truth.

Parents who didn't cuddle their children were probably themselves not touched and held. Some parents are overwhelmed by their own pain and fears they're unable to provide a sense of safety for their children. This leaves the child feeling vulnerable and anxious.

Research supports that many abused children manage to thrive. Kids' brains can change in response to new healthy experiences. No matter what the challenge, many kids cope extremely well with adversity and go on to meet normal developmental expectations. (Note: Coping well is not the same as bouncing back.)

- Reason #1: A tenacious will. (I suggest reading Dave Pelzer's memoirs of childhood abuse: *A Boy Named It; The Lost Boy; A Man Named Dave*.)
- Reason #2: The strong effect of kind, available, caring, trusting, and supportive people (people who encourage, recognize some talent, and nurture their skills) … and faith in God.

God created us with the ability to bring ourselves back from the edge of chaos to reestablish a sense of meaning and independence. If we have a history of childhood abuse, it doesn't have to be our destination or legacy. We can grow up to be powerful advocates and do wonderful work.

If you are victim, hear me: What you have learned, can be unlearned. Lies and false accusations can be un-believed when replaced by the truth! Children are not doomed to repeat the experiences of their parents. This means when you connect with God and immerse yourself in His Word, you will begin to see yourself the way God created you—a royal princess! (1 Peter 2:9)

Every day we have a chance to change our past and our future by reprogramming the present. Remember: it is *never* a minor's responsibility to tell an adult to stop abusing her. That responsibility falls on the adult. Also remember: *Just because someone is unwilling or incapable of loving us, that does not mean we are unlovable.*

† To heal: *write a letter to yourself as a child.* Tell her your heart. Tell her how wonderful she is; that she never deserved to be wounded; that those events don't identify who she is *now*. Reassure her that abuse will no longer run her life; that she is a survivor—*a thriver!* Assure her she can stand up and take charge of her life, overturning all lies and replacing the distortions with Truth.

If You are a Parent

I have three thoughts on this. One, we can't really give to our children what we don't have ourselves. The greatest gift we can give our children is to continue to work on ourselves. As I said before, children learn through imitation. Our greatest opportunity to positively affect each child is to accept and give God's love and to live a godly life.

Second, if our own children have been exposed to abuse, the cycle can be broken. Important factors include having at least one stable relationship during childhood, getting into a good Bible-based church, and getting therapy at some point.[45] Every child must accept the truth that the abuse and violence that happened was not their fault. *There is nothing that child could have done differently that would have led to a different outcome.*

Third, the good news is it's never too late to be a good mom or dad, and to have a positive influence. It's up to you to point your children to God—the only One who can put them back together and strengthen and guide them. He has an incredible plan for their lives too! How does this give you hope for a healthy future?

Ahuva: The Woman at the Well

In John 4:1-42 Jesus introduces us to an unnamed woman, who braved the sun's scorn each day to come to Jacob's well to draw water, all in an attempt to avoid the stares and whispers from the other women. She was a Samaritan—a member of a hated mixed race. (Samaritan's practiced a twisted form of Judaism.) She came always at noon and alone, with her empty jar, a symbol of her life.

One day she sees an unfamiliar face—Jesus. Scripture says that Jesus *had to* go through Samaria (John 4:4-7). Most Jews took the long way to avoid this town. Not Jesus; He was on a mission. He had come to provide salvation for the Samaritans, not annihilate them as His disciples wanted to do (Luke 9:52-55).

Let's not negate this dear lady with the "Samaritan woman" label. Soren Kierkegaard said, "When you label me, you negate me." Let's call her *Ahuva,* which in Hebrew means "beloved."[46]

Ahuva likely thought, *Darn! There's a man at the well today—a Jew! Perhaps he won't notice me. I'll fill my pot quickly and leave.*

This man noticed her. He crossed every boundary and spoke. No respectable Jewish man would talk to a woman, let alone such an outcast like her. Then He asked her for a drink.

Feeling undeserving of His acknowledgment, she reminded Him of her ethnicity. Bracing for rebuke, nothing came from His lips. Instead He gently said, *"If you knew the gift of God and who it is that asks you for a drink, you would have asked him and he would have given you living water."* No one had ever spoken to her before about spiritual thirst so she confused the two kinds of water.

Jesus answered her, *"Everyone who drinks this [well] water will be thirsty again, but whoever drinks the water I give him will never thirst. Indeed, the water I give him will become in him a spring of water welling up to eternal life."* She asked for some of the water. But Jesus redirected her,

"Go, call your husband and come back."

"I have no husband," she replied.

Jesus responded, "You are right when you say you have no husband. The fact is, you have had five husbands, and the man you now have is not your husband" (John 15-18).

Did Ahuva drop her bucket or just her mouth? *How could he have known this?* Jesus saw right into her soul. He already knew every detail about her past before she spoke—and there was no condemnation.

Author and Senior Pastor of Parkview Christian Church, Tim Harlow, wrote, "Why do American pastors always assume this woman was immoral? She was a woman who lived in a culture where she couldn't take care of herself. She had to live with a man in some way. Having five husbands and living with a guy doesn't mean she was immoral. If she had been divorced five times, it was most likely because she had been dumped by her husband five times."[47] The law in those days was pretty lenient for the husband because women were very low on the totem pole and considered a piece of property (see Deuteronomy 24:1-4).

Back then, if you lose your bride-like looks, your husband can say "Adios, you hag!" Not only that, you're considered "defiled." Women had zero rights. A woman couldn't divorce a man if he was "displeasing" or abused her. There was no welfare system, nor could she get a job. Women depended on men to survive. This is why the early church was instructed to care for widows. Some commentators speculate she had been divorced and passed from guy to guy because she couldn't have children—which in those days was a woman's highest value.

I believe this woman was in great emotional pain. Doesn't this change your perspective about Ahuva? Jesus knew her backstory. He gently critiqued her life without crushing her. I doubt very much she felt judged because the Bible is clear that Jesus never condemns anyone. (The combination of grace and truth that Jesus used in this situation is what we experience in our relationship with Him.)

I love this next part. *"The woman said, 'I know the Messiah is coming—the one who is called Christ. When he comes, he will explain everything to us." Then Jesus told her, "I AM the Messiah!"* (vv. 25-26).

Don't miss this: Ahuva was the first person He told that He was the Messiah—the first person! Why didn't He tell the disciples first? Why "the Samaritan woman"? Jesus never makes a wrong choice. He saw right through her. The tribes of northern South Africa have a greeting phrase: *Sawubona,* which literally means "I see you."

This is how Jesus greets us—"Sawubona, my dearest daughter!"

Scripture says that many of the Samaritans from that town believed in Jesus because of her testimony. Psalm 66:16 states, *"Come and listen, all you who fear God, and I will tell you what he did for me."* Despite Ahuva's reputation, many came out to meet Jesus. And He—the Jewish rabbi—hung out with the "dreadful" Samaritans!

Jesus used her story—her broken story to transform many lives. That was His plan all along. He knew from the beginning of time that Ahuva would be the one He'd use to witness to the Samaritans.

Before I was ever conceived, God knew He wanted to use me to write this study and share my story to glorify Him and help you. And before the earth was ever formed, He planned to use you and your story to glorify Him and help others.

German scholar and philosopher Friedrich Nietzsche declared, "He who has a *why* to live for can bear almost any *how.*" Morgan Harper Nichols said, "Tell the story of the mountain you climbed. Your words could become a page in someone else's survival guide."

4

THE WAYS WE RESPOND TO PAIN

You have an unbelievable brain! Did you know it stores every conclusion you make about every experience? And every new experience is treated as reality—until it's instructed to do otherwise. The mind only has access to what it has learned. It can't use what it doesn't know. If you are given only misinformation and lies, then that's all you have access to. Every piece of information is stored with a certain importance attached to it.

It is the mind's job to believe whatever it has stored. To you, its ways are right. This is why you believe you're right and others are wrong even if they don't agree with you. It is for these reasons that we continually use misinformation in trying to process our feelings. Your brain, like my brain, makes decisions based on biased, convoluted and mistaken input. It's true! The more you think negative or scary thoughts, the more brain synapses gets strung together to generate negative scenarios.

A leading Christian psychiatrist, Dr. Timothy Jennings, states in his research that when we consistently believe fear-based lies—for example lies about ourselves, such as, "No one could ever love me," "I'm a bad person," or "I deserve the beatings because I'm a bad wife," or even lies about God, such as, "He is a tyrant and doesn't care about me;" then what happens is our brains get stuck in a survival and fear mode.

Each experience we collect in our brains is tagged with a feeling or feelings and is based on how we see and interpret the experience (called *perception*). Our personal values, judgments, and learned responses are based on these experiences.

Dancing in the Sonshine | 55

When we have a new experience, our brains automatically: Take a snapshot of what we see *(new experience)*, then it finds the *old experience images* in our mind (like puzzle pieces) that *match our new present experience*. The closer the new experience connects to *an existing image*, the more we will *see the new experience* in the same light. If the old existing image was displeasing, the new image will be displeasing.

Take for instance a documentary on a Stone Age Tribe. In one scene, they show the children and adults combing through the hair of the other tribe members, then picking out bugs and eating them delightfully because their collection of old images tells them bugs are *yummy!* For us—not so yummy. Our images tell us to scream if we find bugs in our hair.

For example, Robyn's parents constantly fought "ugly" in front of her *(old image)*. Today when Robyn hears *anyone* raise their voice in conflict *(new image)*, she gets anxious and fearful because the new image ties back to the old image. And, this is why a returning vet hits the ground at the sound of a backfiring vehicle.

When an experience has deeply wounded us, the images associated with that experience, along with the emotions we felt at that time like fear, anxiety, hopelessness, rejection, worthlessness, or not belonging—are forever attached to these images. This can create deadly thinking which takes over and structures our entire world.

Joe called Ashley a "fat ugly pig," not once, but four times. His words offended her greatly. Even when Joe is in a good mood, when Ashley sees Joe walk into the room, or when she thinks of him, the feeling of anger comes over her.

Good news: *Our image brain maps are changeable.* Misconstrued thoughts and feelings can be reshaped. We don't have to be slaves to them. We can develop new healthy ones!

What we need to recognize is our perspective on a particular situation may seem right and logical, but it will always be limited. God's perspective, however, is perfect. And as we continue to get to know Him through His Word, we will begin replacing our error-based perspectives with truth.

† *Reflect on these questions:*
- How does it make you feel to know that you repeatedly use misinformation in trying to process your feelings?
- Can you pinpoint any images which have created deadly thinking?

Post-Traumatic Stress

The past isn't your past if it is still affecting your present. You can try to run from your own wounds, but you'll leave a trail of blood behind. —Kimberly

Have you ever considered that you may living out the hurts of your past because you have PTSD? It's a fact: We live in a traumatic world (John 16:33). We all experience "trauma." It's very common.

If you've been sexually violated or raped, recognize this violation is considered one of the highest factors for the development of PTSD. Symptoms seen in survivors of rape, domestic violence and incest are essentially the same as the symptoms seen in survivors of war. Yet most victims don't recognize they've been through a war. They just think they're crazy. Therapist Linda Graham wrote,

> Few of us will get through an entire lifetime without our resilience being seriously challenged by the pain and suffering inherent in the human condition. None of us is immune to being asked to cope with that we never asked for, with what we deeply, deeply do not want.[48]

Trauma, a.k.a. "Post-Traumatic Stress," is the response to any deeply distressing event that shatters your safe world, so it feels no longer safe. Trauma is a *normal reaction to an overwhelming event or situation that we experience as potentially harmful, that exceeds our ability to cope at the time, and has lasting negative effects.* It is common to experience different kinds of trauma throughout life. It is our cumulative exposure, rather than our experience of one specific event, that has the most impact on our mental, physical and spiritual health.

The letters PTSD stand for "Post-Traumatic Stress Disorder."

Post = After | *Traumatic* = Trauma | *Stress* = Anxiety | *Disorder* = Reaction

The Greek word for "trauma" means "to wound, damage, or defeat." The human body, in an effort to self-preserve and restore a sense of safety, will respond in a variety of typical ways: *trigger, fear, grief, flashback, hyperarousal and hypervigilance, repression, dissociation, or delusions.* And it always affects the family system.

This is the mind's attempt to make sense of a very significant life event. It is a normal way of adapting. *These are all normal responses. You're not crazy—or getting worse!* Interpret each one through eyes of compassion for yourself; not self-blame or craziness.

PTSD is a *deep intrusive injury to the soul.* It may be a big "T" life-threatening, time-limited, "single-blow" event such as the sudden death of a loved one, an assault, being robbed at gunpoint, abandonment, a bad car accident, job loss, terminal illness, terrorism, war, a natural disaster, or discovering you've been videotaped having sex and it's all over the Internet, or you've been conned out of all your savings.

PTSD may be caused by small "t" repeated and/or prolonged events, such as being bullied, criticized, stalked, hit, harassed, screamed at, or rejected. Abusive trauma is not necessarily life threatening but is life-altering—a traumatic perversion of power and distortion of authority.

Experiencing *numerous* small "t" events is more harmful than experiencing one big "T" event, say experts. All of these are traumatic losses, and with the exception of the loss of a loved one, few people receive a lot of condolence or support.

Many are haunted by events that didn't cause them to feel terror, but rather shame, guilt, anger, or resentment. Claudia had been raped 20-years ago. To her, that past memory is still very present. When she gets triggered to think of the incident, it feels to her like it's happening all over again.

Though not all abuse is traumatic, it's *always* damaging and causes suffering. Even if you don't suffer from PTSD, we all have experiences of feeling anxious, fearful, shut off, or thoughts we can't get out of our heads. We don't have to undergo a major trauma to develop symptoms that last for years.[49]

Always remember: Whatever the persistent negative emotion you feel is not the cause of your suffering—*it's the symptom*. The likely cause is an *unprocessed memory*. Wherever we go, whatever we do, thoughts and emotions remain alive in our memory networks waiting to be triggered. These kinds of memories can underlie daily problems and our health in widespread and startling ways.

I don't particularly like the term *Post-Traumatic Stress Disorder*. The word "disorder" implies an illness, disease, or mental problem. I, and many other professionals, believe symptoms stemming from trauma are normal and necessary responses to this kind of personal injury. We call it *Post-Traumatic Stress Injury*—PTSI.

Whatever your PTSI is, it is unique to you and a natural reaction to the serious injury you sustained. In contrast to a "disorder," a stress injury is an emotional wound, able to heal and be transformed.

† In what ways do you relate to the descriptions of PTSI?

Four Levels (Layers) of Trauma

It shocks the brain, stuns the mind, and freezes the body. It overwhelms its unfortunate victims and hurls them adrift in a raging sea of torment, helplessness, and despair. –Peter Levine, PhD

What might Dr. Levine be speaking about? Abuse. *Abuse is trauma* which causes a crisis in a person's life. We know the trauma of abuse makes a woman feel overwhelmed, powerless, and out of control.

The abused usually experience four levels of trauma called "compounded or layered trauma." Think of a layered cake:

- *Layer 1*: The *original trauma*, for example, sexual assault.
- *Layer 2: Secondary wounding* is when loved ones and/or close personal acquaintances do not believe you, or discount, judge, or blame you (called *negative advocates*). Note: Some people blame victims to protect their own sense of safety. Or, a parent may be too sick (emotionally or physically) or powerless to intervene on the child's behalf, is unavailable to help.
- *Layer 3: Society's view of the trauma*, which often holds the victim responsible for what has happened and/or treats her as contaminated or ostracizes her. Also, being treated badly by police, ER staff, or defense attorneys. Then you believe you did something to deserve the assault, adding more stress to the original trauma. Consequently, she is "re-victimized," as each incident adds more hurt on top of the other.
- *Layer 4: We torment ourselves with negative self-talk*. When we believe all the lies and false allegations, we re-abuse ourselves by replaying all those mental tapes over and over again. We suffer deeply and cry, "What wrong with *me*?" instead of "What's wrong with the offender or this relationship?" And, sometimes we say we've had enough. We retaliate and self-protect by becoming abusive too.

Compounded trauma makes us feel alone, so, we tend to keep our emotions to ourselves and isolate, thereby unable to receive necessary support and help. We know that survivors who are believed and supported fare much better than those who are not. The good news is that although the bottom layer cannot be changed, all the other layers can change. We can learn to transform our perceptions.

† Describe how you relate to this these different levels of traumas.

The Injured Brain

Dianna's grandfather raped her at 12-years-old. Today, this past event (whether consciously remembered or not) raises in this 28-year-old woman, *a present-day threat of violation* by her closest, most caring friend—her husband. Dianna stiffens, retracts, and collapses in revulsion when she's cuddled by her husband.

Being cuddled and loved by him brings up all the emotional subject matter Dianna had attached to her rape. She is reacting to the combined triggers of men and touch. When this happens, in her mind she is *confused* between a safe and a dangerous person. When her husband gets intimate, her body and mind go into a survival-based mode assuming danger, even when there is no danger. Like a rag doll, Dianna freezes. When the lovemaking is over, Dianna immediately leaves the room.

A trusted adult violated his position of responsibility by sexually victimizing a child. An adult who was supposed to care for her became the attacker. Dianna learned to mistrust any caring advances; fearful they'd lead to further victimization. Her brain installed the event which was interpreted that sex is dirty, painful, and dangerous.

Decades later, she discovers she doesn't enjoy sex with her husband. She reverts back into 12-year-old Dianna and describes sex as "revolting." Though the adult Dianna believes intellectually that sex is beautiful and safe, she emotionally and physically freezes whenever her husband touches her intimately. Her young brain had installed the image that sex is "icky" which became a key belief. Sadly, a precious child of God who should have been experiencing intimacy and ecstasy with her husband had been robotically reduced to freeze.

What Is Going On?

Why does this happen? Trauma is an injury; a wounding of the brain. It changes brain chemistry and disrupts the way we process information. It affects how we interpret and store the traumatic event. It overrides the brain's alarm system.[50] "It freezes thinking," as Norman Wright says.

When a person is traumatized, the brain is wired to be alert for danger, so she instinctually goes into "survival mode." The instinct is to either *fight, flight,* or *freeze*— "a physiological reaction that occurs in response to a perceived harmful event, attack, or threat to survival."

Trauma causes an increase in the secretion of stress hormones and changes in specific brain structures (the *amygdala* and *hippocampus*) that disrupt normal memory process, resulting in traumatic memories being consolidated and stored differently than non-traumatic memories. We lose all sense of emotions and physical reactions.

Changes in the brain (due to the prolonged effects of *cortisol*—the stress hormone) make it more likely to cement and replay negative, worrisome or distressing memories. This is how traumatic memories get stored, making it harder to learn and store new information.[51]

Another thing we need to recognize is that if we've been adversely wounded or traumatized in the fight, flight or freeze mode, our brain gets stuck in that frozen state. It keeps relaying the negative messages we heard when the event happened such as, "You're not lovable," or "You're a bad/weak person."

Trauma disconnects the left and right sides of the brain. This is why we may have vivid, graphic thoughts about the event, but no emotion. Or, why we experience intense emotions without an actual thought or memory. What is interesting is that when our brain is in this mode—it's not focusing on making new memories—unless those memories will be lifesaving.

Knowing this can help you make sense and normalize your experiences.

PTSI Responses

Pain demands to be felt. –Unknown

Do you ever wonder why some people are "fine" after a trauma and others are not? Somehow their brain managed to process it. With PTSI, no two people have identical reactions, even to the same event. One person feels in control; the other doesn't. The person's childhood attachment history, age, social network, and coping skills have something to do with it.

The type of trauma a person suffers makes a difference. The impact is always based on the severity of *the response* to the event versus the severity of *the event*. The more severe a trauma the more severe its effects. And trauma images may not surface as a conscious memory, but as *emotions, sensations, and bodily responses* long after the event is over. It's physiologically how we're wired.

With a normal experience, the brain processes an experience and turns it into a memory. However, with a big traumatic event the brain can't process it correctly. Our brain wants to protect us from further devastation so it isolates the memories of the event so they're no longer connected with the brain's conscious processing of the experience. One way is called "dissociation," a detachment from reality. It's like these memories get separated and placed in a vault off to the side by themselves (a vertical process).

"Repression" of memories is similar. These memories get pushed down below the surface and stored in the unconscious (a horizontal process). Yet they both silently direct our thoughts and behavior.

Symptoms may lie dormant, only to come up years, even decades later. *Any new event can be unconsciously linked with a separated memory.* We feel a certain way without knowing why: *I'm afraid and I don't know why.*

Fear is normal. When we lose something or someone we value, we can feel disorganized, chaotic, even crazy, which can turn into fear. When the abuse ends, essentially the brain and body doesn't know that. The fears and impressions that registered during the abuse, still registers.

Some "reenact" their trauma called *trauma repetition*. This is when a person (unconsciously) seeks situations or persons that re-create the trauma or abuse experience. This is why many people find themselves in the same kind of abusive situation, with the same type of person, over and over again. Many of us thrive on creating chaos.

Another form of reenactment is to victimize people in the same way others victimized us. For example, a parent who was abused as a child, abuses his/her children. Dr. Patrick Carnes says trauma repetition is "living in the unremembered past and is an effort to bring resolution to the traumatic memory."[52]

Resistant Behavior
Danielle confessed, "At some level I knew what happened (her father had molested her) but I couldn't let myself know, coz then my whole world would have fallen apart."

It's common to lie and argue to others, even to ourselves in order to avoid facing the truth. This happens because the brain will do anything to preserve a sense of a stable self.[53] So, we tend to *distort, rationalize, deceive, blame, disagree/argue, negate, divert/project, reinterpret, dissociate, distance (isolate), repress, or disown.*

Denial and/or *delusion* and/or *minimizing* are very common ways people handle what they cannot handle; a way to keep a toxic experience and the truth of their behavior from surfacing. The truth is just too unbelievable. Instead of a coping mechanism, they revert to a *defense mechanism*.

Our Unconscious Response to Pain

We have great power in the sense that we can choose our habits, but also great responsibility because the habits we have chosen, much more even that the goals we have selected, in the end make us what we are. –Charles Duhigg

Viktor Frankl wrote, "The one thing you can't take away from me is the way I choose to respond to what you do to me."

When someone makes you feel unheard, misunderstood, unloved, guilty, worthless, or shamed, your sense of self is threatened and your brain will work to find ways to feel secure again; to feel in control. *Control* is a means to feel safe and shape reality. Whereas, losing control can induce massive amounts of stress. To avoid this, we become masters at finding ways to mask the painful feelings without speaking our thoughts. Yet interestingly, we choose behaviors that scream, "See my pain!"

The root cause is pain and sin. Somebody has inflicted some type of pain on us. We've been made to feel we're not good enough. A sense of inadequacy and inferiority has been branded on our lives. Our sense of security and significance has been ripped away. Our world has been turned upside down, and nothing seems clear or feels right. This is how we've been shaped.

We choose destructive coping mechanisms because we're lonely, bitter, tormented, frustrated, fearful, shamed, betrayed, lost, lonely, disgusted or grieving. So, we turn to something we think will make us feel better. Our "thing" or person may make us feel better for a short-time, but it always ends up letting us down big-time.

We don't always have control, but we have choices. *The best choice is to examine the cause and process through tough emotions with Jesus and some safe people, and perhaps a qualified counselor.*

The Most Common Coping Methods (a.k.a. Addictions)

A coping method functions as a survival tool by ignoring the pain. Instead of choosing to confront the offender and/or situation, the person instead chooses a coping mechanism behavior as *a way to take back control; to undo the symptoms and memories of a trauma or stressful event; as a way to express their emotions.*

Common techniques are: *Idealization, minimizing, making jokes; addictions* to substances or non-substances; *hostility.* We *rage, criticize,* and are *intolerant* to avoid being attacked ourselves. (Anger and addictions dump chemicals into the body that literally numbs the pain.) Each of these negative coping skills is about hiding, pretending, ignoring, camouflaging—all to protect us from information that would cause us to see ourselves in ways we don't like.

Others are: *outrageousness, smoking, fantasizing, living in the future, people-pleasing, codependency, projection, busyness, perfectionism, compulsiveness, depression/anxiety, sex; excessive: sleeping, plastic surgery, dieting, exercise, tats/body art, working.* Some people use *rage, bullying, control,* and *abuse* to make them feel in control and adequate. The broken thinking goes:

"I'm the attacker who traumatizes—not the one who gets hurt and abused."

Some discover at some point that their toxic feelings can be most effectively stopped by a major jolt to the body—through deliberate inflictions to themselves through: *substance abuse, an eating disorder, and self-harm*. Repetitive self-injury develops most commonly in those whose abuse started early in childhood.[54]

A coping skill can also help us deal with *regret*, that we could have done something to prevent the situation.

We Reap Our Destiny

What I find interesting is our coping mechanisms lead to *biological changes in the brain* → *cravings* → *compulsions* → *repetition* → *deep ruts in thinking patterns* which means they are no longer choices. In other words, our free will gets taken over.

Ralph Waldo Emerson is famous for saying, *"Sow a thought and you reap an action; sow an act and you reap a habit; sow a habit and you reap a character; sow a character and you reap a destiny."*

My primary coping method was food. I began by *choosing* to diet to deal with the anxiety I felt over gaining 15 pounds and my dad's fat-shaming tactics. But soon it got out of control and became a compulsion; then a deadly eating disorder, taking away all free will leading to bondage. I know now I was trying to regulate difficult feelings. Bingeing was a way of distracting me from those feelings; purging a way to feel in control of my body. Being a small size gave me a sense of security.

God has a different plan. *He doesn't ask that we stop craving but rather we crave something different—Him.* He is the one who break the chains of bondage which leads to peace and calm. We must make the decision to lay our troubles in His hands and know that He will take care of the situation—His way and in His time. This is called surrender and faith—faith in His promise: *"I am your God and will take care of you until you are old and your hair is gray. I made you and will care for you; I will give you help and rescue you"* (Isaiah 46:4).

† What battle with a coping mechanism do you need God to fight for you today? Give Him the room to work without trying to seize control.

Every Human's Soul Hole

At the end of the movie *Wizard of Oz,* Glenda the Good Witch tells Dorothy she could have gone home any time. Dorothy questions her, "Why didn't you tell me that before?" Glenda replies, "Because you wouldn't have believed me. You've had the power all along. You had to learn it for yourself." What do we need to know?

The central theme in Genesis 1 and 2 is the interrelationship of the Lord God with His creation, Adam and Eve, our original parents. Chapter 2 ends with a short but striking account of the perfection of the first human beings. Then Chapter 3 opens with an account of their degradation and ruin, called "the Fall." As a result, mankind lost their perfect relationship with God. Their minds darkened (Ephesians 4:18). From that day forward, every baby inherited a sinful nature (called "original sin").

Psychiatrist M. Scott Peck, offered his perspective in "Addiction: The Sacred Disease." Dr. Peck believes, as the majority of Christians do, that at birth humans become separated from God (due to original sin). People report feeling empty and refer to it as "a hole in the soul." They sense something is missing, but don't know what it is. At a point in their lives these sensitive souls stumble across an object which makes them feel better—a soul stuffer, like alcohol. Dr. Peck pointed out the alcoholic is really thirsty for the Holy Spirit.[55]

Everybody worships something.

Society has us believing that only more of what it offers will satisfy: a bottle of booze, Facebook and Instagram, cheesecake, a couple of pills, a higher paying job, the perfect man, designer accessories, an educational degree, a pack of smokes, breast implants. Some people have an "Apple-shaped hole" in their heart that only a new iPhone can fill. These things become our default settings.

The famous Sophia Loren once said in an interview that she had everything—awards, money, marriage—but "in my life there is an emptiness impossible to fulfill."

Saint Augustine said, "Because God has made us for Himself, our hearts are restless until they rest in Him." Whether we realize it or not, deep inside we all feel "something" is missing. Our need to be filled up is God-given because God created us to be overfilled by Him. We are designed to hold Him as the object of our deepest affections. When we don't, a hole in our soul is exposed. We can't stand for the hole to be empty so we stuff it with all sorts of things which become the Lord of our lives. Yet we are never satisfied because only God can fill us sufficiently.

Our view of life says everything is to be evaluated on whether it satisfies *my* desires and makes *me* whole. We devour the bait because our souls are hungry for a connection to God, an alignment with the Holy Spirit, and a union with Jesus Christ.

Time and again, the Bible speaks about God's promises to the hungry—to those of us with a huge soul-hole. God *"satisfies the thirsty and fills the hungry with good things" (Psalm 107:9).* God Almighty wants you to enter His promise land.

Step out in faith when God asks you to bury your other gods—those things that rival His rightful place in your soul. The truth is, only He has the power, and the desire, to give you a better and healthier life. How does this make you feel?

The Good News

The good news is, *this cycle can be reversed when we choose to saturate our minds with the truth and reflective insight.* The brain will begin to regrow neural pathways and forge new connections. We know that when a person has a strong desire to change and learn new things, their work leads to astonishing brain changes.

As we've learned, our brains change with *everything* we experience, whether it's good or bad. Our brains—young and old—have the ability to rewire and heal themselves when we learn and remember new things, called brain *plasticity* or *neuroplasticity* (*neuro* = brain cells; *plastic* = changed/altered.) This includes the development of healthy activities or an addiction.

A neuroplastic brain makes it possible to recover from the damage of trauma. The trauma of pain and betrayal can set the stage for *post-traumatic growth* (James 1:2-4). Trauma *and* transformation can co-exist; grief *and* hope can co-exist. Something traumatic can lead to great growth (Romans 8:28). The traumatic event will always be part of your life—but, it doesn't have to be the center of it!

Yale physician, Kate Wheeling wrote, "As soon as something breaks, tears, or malfunctions within us, the instructions in our cells begin to supervise repairs." This is encouraging.

I'd like to paraphrase it to say: "As soon as something breaks, tears, or malfunctions within us, the Holy Spirit in us begins to supervise repairs." God living in us and working in us is makes transformative neuroplasticity possible.

A Supernatural Brain Encounter

Did you know the moment you encounter God, or the idea of God, your brain begins to change?[56] Brain scientists (neuroscientists) have found that when you contemplate God long enough, something surprising happens in the brain—the neural functioning begins to change. Brain imaging confirms that *what you believe about God changes your brain—either positively or negatively*.

Listen to this: Scientists have discovered that when we begin to contemplate something as complex and mysterious as God and the big questions in life, we have incredible bursts of activity firing up in different parts of the brain ... and we grow and heal. When prayer is added, many health benefits have been found, including greater length of life.[57]

It has been found that *12 minutes* of daily focused prayer over an 8-week period can change the brain to such an extent that it can be measured on a brain scan.[58] Therefore, even though toxic thoughts can cause brain damage, *prayer can reverse that damage and cause the brain and body to thrive.*

The greatest brain and lifestyle improvements occurred when participants meditated specifically on a loving God for at least 12 minutes per day for 66 days.[59] This is because our brains have been designed to meditate on truth, which enables detachment from emotions like fear and shame. No fitness, self-help, or medical program can do this! Making a commitment to pray and meditate on Bible verses and testimonies that focus on God's love and goodness *is the prescription for change.* It can lower overall levels of stress while increasing cognitive alertness and empathy.

Steve Arterburn, chairman of *New Life Ministries*, stated that research supports that people who spend at least 4 out of 7 days of the week in God's Word experience *significant transformational change.*

Meditate means to "reflect on." The Hebrew word is *habah* which means "to be preoccupied with; be absorbed with." This doesn't have the meaning of glancing at something. It means to reflect deeply and ponder what each verse means. Get personal. What is God saying to *you*? Grapple with it; study it; visualize it as reality—for 12 minutes.

I'll warn you that after 5 or so minutes you'll think you've seen all there is to see. I challenge you to keep going. Write down at least 12 things (1 per minute) you see or learn from the verse. It will change your spiritual life and relationship with God. This is harnessing the power of God's living Word.

God tells us in the Bible to meditate on His Words day and night (Joshua 1:8). So, what's 12 minutes? The end of the verse reads, *"Then you will be prosperous and successful."* Who doesn't want this?

A Different Coping Mechanism

Anything I wanted I took and did not restrain myself from any joy. I even found great pleasure in hard work. This pleasure was, indeed, my only reward for all my labors. But as I looked at everything I had tried, it was all so useless, a chasing of the wind, and there was nothing really worthwhile anywhere.

—Solomon, speaking in Ecclesiastes 2:10-11

Many professionals suggest changing to a different behavior, as in "behavior modification." The problem is this doesn't allow people to be internally transformed, but rather pushes them to merely conform. We can't merely modify our behavior because the underlying pain still exists, and we'll eventually switch to another behavior, like musical chairs. We must make the decision to deal with the underlying pain.

Lamentations 3:40 states, *"Instead, let us test and examine our ways. Let us turn back to the LORD."* No matter how religious or spiritual we think we are, our behaviors are always capable of sidetracking our love for God. The more we can understand how enslavement happens, the more we'll be able turn the opposite way—back towards God, the Creator of freedom.

Most people finally realize they'll never stay sober until they find the reasons they became an alcoholic or people-pleaser or bulimic, for example. Coming to terms with the pain and changing thinking patterns is the place to start, which is the goal of this study. What helps many people stay sober is the work they do on themselves with God, professionals, support groups, and trusted friends.

When addiction researchers scanned recovered addict's brains, quite often they found that the parts related to cravings still light up when the person sees or imagines their "favorite desirable thing." But—the part of the brain that says, "Do it!" is overridden by new activity in the brain region relating to self-discipline and inhibitions.[60]

Painful and traumatic experiences can tempt you to either run to God or run away from God. A crisis will not last forever. A recurring phrase (453 times) in the Bible is *"it came to pass."* I say run to God.

Restoration takes time, so be patient with yourself and Him. God said *"… no weapon forged against you will prevail" (Isaiah 54:15)*. No one is a lost cause to God. He is faithful to His promises today just as much He was to the people in biblical times.

God promises to guide us through a time of crisis and change: *I will be with you; and when you pass through the rivers, they will not sweep over you. When you walk through the fire, you'll not be burned; the flames will not set you ablaze" (Isaiah 43:2). The LORD hears his people when they call to him for help. He rescues them from all their troubles (Psalm 34:17).*

† How confident do you feel about your level of readiness for change?

1	2	3	4	5	6	7	8	9	10
Not confident									Extremely confident

Healing Coping Strategies

Dr. Manuel J. Smith wrote,

> Not only is it natural to expect that we will have problems in living, it is also natural to expect that we all can cope adequately with these problems. If we did not have the inherited ability to cope, human beings would have died out a long time ago.

Express Your Emotions

How do you feel? If I asked you this question how would you answer? "Fine." That's a typical safe answer. You're most likely not trying to be evasive. It's likely an honest answer; your way of saying, "I don't know." If you grew up denying or repressing your emotions, it's likely a habit.

Dr. Dan Allender wrote, "Emotions are like messengers from the front lines of the battle zone. Our tendency is to kill the messenger. But if we listen carefully, we will learn how to fight the war successfully."

I learned in my healing journey that an eating disorder becomes a wordless substitute for the person's negative feelings she has toward people who have wronged, ignored, slighted and taunted her. At the same time, she is also trying desperately to coax others to pay attention to her needs, which she doesn't or can't verbalize.

I had to learn to put words to my emotions. Some people have learned to "blow off steam" by punching a pillow or throwing a soft object. Experts say these methods don't work. They only reinforce feelings of anger and anxiety. Start to practice putting words to your emotions.

To face deep-seated feelings can be one of the most scary and painful aspects of healing. Yet it's one of the first rewards—releasing the pain and pressure. It's a way to unlearn unhealthy behavior patterns and raise your level of self-esteem. I suggest you take time throughout each day to think critically about your interactions. Ask yourself: *How do I feel about this?*

This may sound foreign, even scary to you; please hear me. There is *power* in admitting to and *talking about traumatic and stressful events*. Even one abuse experience can be traumatic. We need to find a way to express what happened. Being able to articulate our experiences through either speaking of a specific incidence, telling our story, or writing about it quite often provides a powerful way for overcoming pain. The process itself helps us make sense of our experiences. "Feel it" so you can "heal it." We do need to be a good judge about who we can share our stories with.

Consider Journaling

For many survivors, saying in words how we feel is too difficult. Consider writing. Writing is an emotional outlet, and form of prayer that does something no other form of expression can do. One counselor calls it *taking out our emotional trash*. Naming our beliefs and writing about distressing events in detail, is the only kind of writing that clinically has been associated with improved health.[61]

Numerous sources report that 20-minute writing sessions about emotional topics, on consecutive days, reduced PTSD symptoms, depression, and anxiety after two weeks.[62] You don't have to be a writer to do this or buy a fancy journal. Use the "Feeling Wheel" in Appendix A as a guide to help you express yourself.

I encourage you write to God for 15 to 20-minutes a day about any painful or traumatic memories. Express your fears, worries, and difficult experiences. Many people find they begin writing about things the hadn't consciously thought about for years. They probe deeply because writing and God are safe. Tell Him how you feel.

God has a wonderful way of helping us call up the past without us becoming overwhelmed by those memories. He can enter into our anguish and interject His own pain and perspective into our writing. You can voice your disapproval of what God allowed to happen. If you're annoyed at God, tell Him so. It's a powerful way to validate your experiences and emotions.

Most women come to see their situations differently through writing. The benefit is you can begin to find self-forgiveness and then shift any guilt and self-blame onto the real offender. Describe how the types of abuse affected you: Talk about all the losses you discovered, coping mechanisms, relationships, and any self-sabotaging behavior. You can write about the person you want to be, and how you want your life to go. Don't be afraid to express regrets.

Talk about the things you wish had ended differently; the unrealized hopes, dreams, and expectations; what was said or not said; things done or not done; the fences you want mended. Listen to your body and record any physical sensations.

You may decide you want to write a letter to your abuser and not send it. This can be very therapeutic. Akin to journaling would be painting or drawing or arts n' crafts. Instead of words, you use art to express yourself. The same with music.

Use journaling to understanding the "why."

- How do I want to be loved? How do I want to be known?
- What am I afraid for others to know about me?
- What wounds and lies cause me to believe I'm not choose-able?

Use journaling to figure out the "hidden agenda" behind your coping mechanisms.

- What do you hope to accomplish with this behavior?
- How does it make your life more satisfying?
- What affect do you have on others by using this behavior?
- What would happen if you gave up your coping mechanism?
- What fears do you have giving it up?
- How will you feel once you are free?

Consider Anonymity
Many people feel safer revealing themselves where their identity is unknown. This is why online support and recovery groups are so popular. Revealing things that we've kept secret for years in the company of strangers helps many find others with whom they can share their "real self" with. This is often a first step of feeling accepted. Through this venue, we can get comfortable bridging ourselves from writing to speaking. Like any other venue, you need to vet whether the group is safe or not for you.

Connect with Safe and Healthy People
I've been around now for quite a while. I remember the way we lived a few decades ago, and today is vastly different than it was then. Back then, men and women had a much wider access to social networks churches, community groups, afterschool clubs and groups and unions. People were part of a larger world; they were connected. Today, with our high level of mobility and our focus on technology and ourselves/consumerism, we tend to be far more socially isolated.

This means any one person can take on enormous influence if we're isolated from other healthy sources. A partner or parent can come to be the sole source of emotional and material support. As a result, we focus all our needs for love and approval on these relationships, which ultimately define who we are.

If we lived in a more traditional culture, we'd have a larger range of emotional connections to help us see truth. Today we need to reach out to other healthy individuals and groups. We need safe places and people to express our emotions to—to cry with and to express our justified anger.

Experts state that talking through experiences with others allows us to convert upsetting and traumatic experiences into *post-traumatic growth*.[63] It helps us construct the meaning of our injury.

The other thing talking it out does is create *vulnerability* which means we're no longer terrified of our past. I love Brené Brown's definition of *vulnerability*. She wrote,

> Vulnerability is based on mutuality and requires boundaries and trust. It's not oversharing, it's not purging; it's not indiscriminate disclosure. It is about sharing our feelings and experiences with people who have earned the right to hear them. Being vulnerable and open is mutual and an integral part of the trust-building process. We don't lead with, "Hi, my name is Brené and here's my darkest struggle. That's not vulnerability. That may be desperation or woundedness or co-dependency or even attention-seeking, but it's not vulnerability. Sharing appropriately, means sharing with people with whom we've developed relationships that can bear the weight of our story. The result: increased connection and trust.
>
> We have found ways to protect ourselves from vulnerability, from being hurt, diminished, and disappointed. We put on armor; we used our thoughts, emotions, and behaviors as weapons; and we learned how to make ourselves scarce, even disappear. Now as adults we realize that to live with courage, purpose, and connection—to be the person whom we long to be—we must again be vulnerable. *We must take off the armor, put down the weapons, show up, and let ourselves be seen.*[64]

As people are there for us, we need to be there for others. Empathizing with people's stories help them feel they don't have to conquer their struggles and heartaches alone. This is because God designed us to connect and bear one another's burdens (Galatians 6:2).

† Think about these questions:
- What are your core beliefs about being vulnerable and sharing your story? (For example, do you believe you honor the people in your

circle by sharing your pain and allow them into your experience. Or do you feel like you're dumping on them; putting them on the spot?)
- What fears do you have about sharing your pain?

Meditate on Scripture for 12 Minutes a Day

The beginning of feeling lovable, of being able to love and experience belonging, begins by believing you are so loved by God and belong to Him. What do these verses mean to you?

- *Love:* "For *God so loved the world [you]* that *he gave* his one and only Son, that whoever believes in him shall not perish but have eternal life" *(John 3:16). See also: Romans 8:35-39.*
- *Attachment:* "Through the power of the Holy Spirit *who lives within us [you]*, carefully guard the precious truth that has been entrusted to you" *(2 Timothy 1:14);* "Don't you know that you yourselves are God's temple and that *God's Spirit lives in you?" (1 Corinthians 3:16). See also: John 14:23; 15:4.*
- *Love & Attachment:* "This is how *God showed his love* among us: He sent his one and only Son into the world that *we might live through him*" *(1 John 4:9). See also Isaiah 43:1.*
- *Be Known:* "O LORD, you have searched me and *you know me*" *(Psalm 139:1—read the entire Psalm 139);* "I *[God] knew you* before you were formed within your mother's womb ..." *(Jeremiah 1:5).*
- *Be Chosen:* "You did not choose Me but *I chose you" (John 15:16);* "*You are a chosen people ... God's special possession (1 Peter 2:9).*

Other Suggestions

Tackle the triggers. It's important to specifically identify triggers and avoid them. Most often, triggers are situations and/or emotions we're not aware of. Document episodes in order to look for trigger patterns. Ask yourself the *who, what, when, where, how,* and *why* questions:

- Who is with you when you're tempted ...?
- What happened right before you did this behavior?

- When and where are you most tempted?
- How do you usually feel when you're most tempted?
- Why do you think this happens?

Use positive distractions: Explore your reservoir of talents and interests. If you have a desire to paint and draw, or do arts and crafts, do it. Exercising and walking are good for you. Listen to music, sing, and/or play an instrument. Pray and read the Bible. Go to church. Talk to family and friends. Take a self-defense class. Get a pet or play with a pet. Put together a puzzle. Cook a meal; clean your house. Watch a funny movie. Get a massage. Take a warm bubble bath. Practice the self-care exercises.

Create a new sense of control. We can carve out areas where we do have control. For example, binge eating is a very common coping mechanism. When craving a particular food, instead of constantly telling yourself "no" create a situation where you can say yes. Tara called herself an "eating machine." She decided to create a chart that had a list of the foods she could eat (wise choices). As she put it, "This eating machine could eat all day as long as the food was on the chart." Tara's solution gave her back a sense of control.

You may find yourself mourning the loss of your trusted and beloved coping strategy. In every change experience, something may be taken away, but we are being given something we didn't have before. You will come to celebrate the alternative—to feel empowered with the knowledge that you can keep yourself safe and healthy. And as you move forward through this study and learn to challenge false beliefs and replace them with truth, you should find it easier to let go of your "old friend."

You can do this. I'm proof! We're partners with the living God in this. God gives us intelligence and abilities to complete this work—with Him. He promises a *co-creating partnership*.

5

Is Your Love Tank Empty?

My (Kimberly) weekends as a young adult were spent in bars looking for Mr. Right, followed by nursing hangovers and my dignity. I cannot count how many times I woke up with a strange man, staring at the ceiling, pretending to be loved and needed and desired.

> *Will he want to get to know me; perhaps ask me to spend the day with him? Or is he simply another "smooth operator?" Will he, like the others, promise to call only to dismiss me? Might he actually want to start a relationship—a meaningful love relationship my soul craves?*

Then this situation triggered old thoughts and feelings. I thought about the other guys I'd met at bars; about how nasty and shaming those experiences had been. Being repeatedly rejected fueled cynical and destructive feelings: *I can't believe I'm in this place again. I feel used, abused, and embarrassed. I hate myself. This keeps happening because I'm bad.*

I kept hoping that each new encounter would *the* one, only to be disappointed when I'd get exactly what I'd previously gotten.

In our desperate search to find an intimate mate, we get into relationships we don't truly want to be in, but the acceptance factor is so great. We jump through hoop after hoop to be accepted and loved. We delude ourselves into thinking sex will motivate a guy to "be there" for us.

I always had to have a man in my life. It was a kind of validation I wasn't as worthless as I thought I was. I believed, like so many women, that any kind of relationship is better than no relationship.

It's better to settle for crumbs.

I learned as a teen that guys want sex. So, if you're going to be in any kind of relationship with a guy, give him sex. Sex was inevitable, whether I desired it or not. If I received no sexual response, it felt like rejection because I learned my only value was as a sexual object.

My heart broke as I was betrayed time after time. I'd feel like I got punched in the gut, but unconsciously I believed I couldn't do any better. There's actually a scientific explanation. There are areas of the brain designed to create deep bonds between individuals to ensure their wellness. When those types of relationships are not present, or when a significant relational break occurs—by either rejection, abandonment, or a type of abuse, *the brain registers the emotional pain the same way it registers the pain of a physical injury.*

† In what ways do you see yourself in this description and/or in my story?

"I Only Wanna Be with You!"

As we spend time with our mate, our brains start to release another neurochemical called *oxytocin*, nicknamed "the love hormone." Unlike the quick high of dopamine, oxytocin is subtler and sticks around longer, leading to a deeper attachment.

Oxytocin is also called the "superglue hormone." It is powerful. It's the same hormone that bonds a mother to her newborn baby. For example, if a young woman becomes physically close and hugs a guy, oxytocin will be released and trigger the bonding process. This creates a greater desire to be near him and, most significantly, trust him. If he then wants to escalate the relationship, it becomes harder for her to say no because oxytocin extends the feelings of pleasure.[65]

Oxytocin triggers an involuntary process that cannot distinguish between a hook up or a one-night stand or a committed relationship. When we bond with another human being, the unbonding process often causes great emotional damage and pain. We all have neural cells around the heart that can feel the rupture of disconnection; it's a feeling of having a "hole in the heart."[66]

Whenever a breakup takes place there is often pain, or disappointment, or confusion because the bond has been broken.[67]

Sara said, "I'm an adult now—26 years-old. I never had a relationship with a guy last very long. They always seem to end once the sex is over. And now that I'm married, I don't get why people think sex is so great."

There is a reason Sara feels this way: The inability to bond after multiple sexual encounters is a consequence. She no longer has the ability to bond to her husband. It is very much like tape that loses its stickiness after being applied and removed multiple times.[68]

† How do you relate to oxytocin and Sara's story?

Our Love Tanks

Mother Teresa advocated, "The most terrible poverty is loneliness, and the feeling of being unloved." She felt the greatest problem on earth was being unloved. She said that in the West, we experience poverty of the spirit, loneliness, and being unwanted.[69]

Most human suffering is related to love and the loss of it. Science proves *humans are wired for love*. Every heart cries, *"Love me! I need to be loved and noticed."* Deep down, we all want to know, *"Am I lovable and beautiful? Am I good?"* Sadly, damaging and unequipped parents, and this culture, have a way of implying, "There's nothing about you that is beautiful or lovable," thereby creating a great source of pain.

Do you realize you have a "love tank" that needs refueling as frequently as your car does? Many professionals refer to our basic need for love as a need to fill our love tanks. The first people who must fill them are our parents. The problem is, if parents aren't keeping each other's love tanks replenished, they usually can't fill their child's tank adequately (meaning their parenting skills or absence comes short of what we need).

When our cry for love and acceptance is ignored or abused, then the potential for any destructive behavior springs up because it distracts us from the pain of feeling unloved. Since we don't have a clear picture of what "normal" godly love is, we end up wandering down Heartbreak Road.

When our love tanks aren't filled, self-worth deteriorates, and impacts how we relate to others, even how we feel about God. Yet, *feeling* unloved has nothing to do with our worth—we just interpret it this way. How we see ourselves today (our sense of self-esteem, self-worth, self-image) and the quality of our interactions (our beliefs about relationship), are all strongly influenced by our parents, particularly our mothers.

If we were never hugged, then we have the tendency to run to the first guy who will embrace and stay with us. *Don't leave. Be with me forever.* We become willing to suffer the consequences just to get a hug, a kiss, and hear the words which confirm we're lovable, important, and beautiful. *Please love me!* This is one way we get into trauma-bonded relationships so easily.

† How full is your love tank?

Our Foundation to Love and to be Loved

Jennine asked, "Since I've never in my life had a full love tank, nor experienced real love, how can I ever love someone?" Given Jennine's family dysfunction, we might say she doesn't have the foundation or ability to love as God created her to love—or does she? The Bible tells us: *"God is love ... God lives in us, and his love is brought to full expression in us" (1 John 4:8; 12).*

- If you are a believer, you know God, who is the definition of Love.
- And Love (God) lives in you and has poured His love into you.
- Therefore, you have the ability to love another person and to be loved the way God created you to love and be loved.

It's easy to say all this, and harder to grasp. The clincher is: We need to first learn to love God and allow Him to love us. This is our love-foundation.

✝ How does this sit with you? Can you step forward in faith and love as God desires you to love? Explain.

Mommy and Daddy "Holes"

"You can't have that. You're fat!" Dad snatched the plate of food away as I (Kimberly) reached for seconds. "I bet you weigh 150 pounds. Get on the scale and let's see," he barked.

The humiliation crushed my soul. *If my dad—whose approval I desperately seek—thinks I'm fat, then everyone else does.* There is no opinion as important as our parents. What they say, we believe. Consequently, I allowed my dad's opinions, throughout my life, to control my thoughts, feelings, and actions. His words made me feel I wasn't good enough or desirable.

This particular event was the trigger that led me into the abyss. The combination of childhood events, the feelings of unworthiness, combined with fear and loneliness, triggered my eating disorder.

You see, I never felt attractive or that I belonged growing up. My classmates nicknamed me Bozo, after the clown. I was always comparing myself to others and coming up short. Add to this that my dad disapproved of all fat people, which too our culture enforces. I always felt I wasn't pretty enough or thin enough; just wasn't enough.

What started as a diet, and a quest for love and acceptance, ended up being a 20-year battle with bulimia, substance abuse, and promiscuity. I lived a double life which looked pretty good to outsiders. I became a master at lying and faking it; a pro at hiding behind designer clothes. I developed unhealthy emotional attachments and measured my self-worth by how a guy—any guy—felt about me in the moment.

These were the lengths I'd go to feel better about myself. Yet, I was so ashamed and worked diligently to keep this secret my entire life. I mean, things like this don't happen to people like me!

Unbeknownst to me, I had both a *daddy hole* and a *mommy hole*—a craving for love, affection, attention; basic emotional needs I didn't receive from my parents. This, I believe, is the clincher: Neither parent took the time to get to "know" me. Instead, I had to conform to their ways.

You see, *to know me is to love me.* What resulted in my adult life was an insatiable "hole." I say a hole because having unavailable parents permanently alters our world. We form views of ourselves, of relationships, of family, even of God, based on our parents' example. Whatever happened in childhood, helped forge who we are today. Thus, counselor's offices **today** are filled with people desperately searching for a mom or dad—usually in all the wrong places.

✝✝✝

There is no question that parental absences, either physically and/or emotionally, brings on serious consequences. Today I know that my parent's lack of involvement didn't help me grow up; not until Jesus came into my life. I stayed a little girl emotionally. All the struggles I experienced as a young adult were directly related to the emotional distance I experienced within my family. A secondary factor in my immaturity was alcohol abuse. The pain and turmoil eventually found respite in ED, my **e**ating **d**isorder.

How a parent responds to our basic needs tells us how important and valuable we are to them, which builds the foundation of our self-worth and self-image. Any psychologist will tell you the most damaging and debilitating betrayal a child can experience is betrayal or the lack of "blessing" by one or both parents.

Jasmin Lee Cori, author of *The Emotionally Absent Mother* and *Healing from Trauma* stated that "good" parental messages say or imply love for the child.[70] How many of these messages did you get from your parents?

- *I'm glad that you're here*—Tells the child she is wanted.
- *I see you*—Being seen is being known.

- *You are special to me*—Tells her she is valued; provides affirmation that she's precious and delightful.
- *I respect you*—Supports her uniqueness and doesn't try to control.
- *I love you unconditionally*—There's nothing you can do to lose my love; You don't have to earn my love; You can be yourself.
- *Your needs are important to me*—You can turn to me for help.
- *I'm here for you and will make time for you*—You can count on me.
- *I'll keep you safe*—I'll protect you.
- *You can rest in me*—I will soothe and comfort you.

† Describe your emotional response to this list and/or my story.

Mommy Holes

If someone said to you, "You're so much like your mom," how would that make you feel? When I was asked this question, I felt 50/50. My mom has a gentle and sweet spirit, but she wasn't a nurturer. Throughout my childhood she appeared disconnected and absorbed elsewhere. She never seemed tuned into my emotional states, nor seemed to care.

Here's the clincher: We learn patterns of intimacy, relating, separation; how to handle failure and troublesome emotions, expectations, grief and loss—from Mom. How we were mothered and how we responded to that mothering determines our emotional development. What we learned in our relationship with our mom deeply affects every aspect of our adult life.

A Swedish study found that even when a mother works outside the home and Dad is the primary caretaker, babies still strongly prefer to be with Mom, due to early bonding behaviors.[71] (*Mother* can refer to an adoptive mother, grandmother, step-mom, or caretaker who takes on a caring, nurturing, protective role in the baby's life.)

Consequently, I suppressed my emotions and turned to some deadly coping mechanisms. I know now Mom loved me but has been limited in her ability to express it. I believe she was under-mothered and unsupported herself, and so she became more focused on her own needs. What I find interesting is she has never really shared any stories from her past.

Many of us have a mommy hole which began in infancy. Psychologists believe "disrupted" or "impaired attachments" (like neglect, detachment, abandonment) or "dismissive attachments" (being uncomfortable with closeness and strong emotions) in a child's life is a key factor in why so many feel unloved. Many of us learned to take unacceptable treatment from others in order to try to prevent feelings of rejection, aloneness and abandonment.

Attachment is often described as a strong bond or feeling of love for someone, usually the parents. A baby's feeling of attachment, or lack of it, is pretty much set by the time she is 1-years-old. Without those secure attachments, the baby/child lacks the tools required to function as a healthy individual. As an adult, she is prone to soothe her basic God-given need for love, attachment, and approval through destructive ways.[72]

In healthy situations, when a mother is loving, nurturing, and attuned, we securely attach; we learn we are loved and lovable. That sense of being lovable—worthy of affection and attention, of being seen and heard—becomes the bedrock on which we build our earliest sense of self and worth. But for one-third of the population who doesn't attach securely, myriads of problems can occur.[73]

Because she is able to observe and feel emotional clues, a baby girl actually incorporates her mother's nervous system into her own. Jennifer's nervous system had imprinted the stress-filled, unsafe reality of her mother's early life, therefore, people seemed unreliable and threatening. Compare that to Kylie's brain circuits, which had incorporated a nurturing, safe mom, therefore, people appeared trustworthy and safe to her.[74]

Dr. Sue Gerhardt stated in her book, *Why Love Matters*, the stress response is mediated by the hormone *cortisol*, and insecurely attached children have too much of it circulating. High levels of cortisol have been associated with eating disorders, alcoholism, and anxiety, as well as damaging the parts of the brain responsible for retrieving information and thinking clearly.[75] The same thing happens if we grow up in families with boundary problems. Bingo! This helped me understand myself better. Even though I was never physically or sexually abused by a family member, there weren't any verbal or behavioral signs that said "I love you."

Insecurely attached children generally lack the ability to form strong bonds with others. For me this meant I was never taught by Mom to connect with other females. So, I looked for a guy to meet *all* of my needs. I never had true girlfriends to help meet some of my "girl" needs. My need for connection was always superimposed upon a guy—who eventually dumped me for being too "needy."

What we must realize is that young children don't have the perspective to understand all the factors that influence their parent's behavior. They mistakenly believe that when others avoid, abandon, or hurt them, it's because they are bad and unlovable. *Mommy, this happened because of me.* This isn't necessarily a conscious feeling.

† With Jesus, use this format to identify your Mommy losses.

Ways My Mom Let Me Down	*"Stuff" and Emotions I Struggle with Today*

Babies Absorb their Parents' Stress and Pain

Scientists have confirmed that a woman's nutritional condition, psychological states and emotional tendencies do in fact influence the predispositions of the children she gives birth to. Such susceptibilities are low-self-esteem and self-worth; anxiety and depression.

Rose had felt afraid, guilty, and unloved during her pregnancy which generated negative thinking, feelings and actions. Her daughter indicated that she has always felt a sense of being unloved, unwanted and unworthy, even though she could never tie a specific experience to her feelings.

Researchers have detected that when a baby perceives any threat through her senses, such as loud, angry voices in the next room, her brain goes on alert. Her heart pumps, her breath becomes rapid and shallow; she sweats, and oxygen rushes to her limbs in an involuntary fight-or-flight response. But since Baby can't fight or flee, she moves into a freeze state; sort of numb. This is a trauma state.

Once the brain has become hypervigilant to danger, it's more easily triggered: the *amygdala* stays on high alert to access what's coming next. And when it detects danger in Baby's environment, her little brain quickly goes into a heightened state of hypervigilance, called "kindling."

From this point on, it takes only a small spark or trigger for Baby's brain to burst into a firestorm of reactivity, releasing a sudden blaze of stress hormones and chemicals. Exposure to stress for any baby is like laying kindling on a fire. The person who experiences chronic early trauma is much more susceptible to later reactivity to stressful events.[76]

This process can even begin prenatally. The right brain is the first to develop in the womb, and it carries the nonverbal communication between mothers and infants. Worse, when children get the womb message that they're unwanted or unwelcome, they'll quite often have difficulties finding their way in life.

Healing a Mommy Hole

Part of the healing process is *taking the mask off Mom* and viewing her life story and the forces that shaped her. My mom was adopted and may not have securely attached to her own birth and/or adoptive mother. Add to that, in her "traditional" generation it was expected for a woman to be a mother (which she admitted years later she really didn't want to be). It was a father's role to be the provider, which my dad did well.

I don't have any memories of being held, being looked at with loving eyes, or being emotionally cared for during important years. Nor does my mother have any such memories. Mom and I both grew up intellectually believing we were loved, but not feeling loved by our mothers. It wasn't until Jesus came into both of our lives that we learned to connect with each other and restore our relationship. We have a different kind of relationship today; we're friends.

Joel 2:25 came alive: *"The LORD says, "I will give you back what you lost to the swarming locusts, the hopping locusts, the stripping locusts, and the cutting locusts."* The locusts represent the various losses in our lives. God will provide. He can be mother, and He will put others in our lives to fill in the holes.

We can Attach to Our Heavenly Mother

You may wonder how one mother can fulfill so many important tasks. No one human being can completely, so, we turn to our heavenly Mother—God. Think about this: Why would the Creator of the universe come down to earth as a man and be driven to die? For the same reason a healthy mother would drop everything for the sake of her child.

Most of us are familiar with God's masculine, fatherly characteristics, but are less aware that the Bible contains many female images of God:

- Genesis 1:27: *In the image of God he created them; male and female.*
- Isaiah 49:15: *Can a mother forget the baby at her breast and have no compassion on the child she has borne? Though she may forget, I [God] will not forget you!*
- Isaiah 66:13: *As a mother comforts her child, so will I [God] comfort you …*
- Hosea 13:8: *Like a bear robbed of her cubs, I [God] will attack them and rip them open.*
- Matthew 23:37: *O Jerusalem … how often I [Jesus] have longed to gather your children together, as a hen gathers her chicks under her wings, but you were not willing.*

Fortunately, we have a second chance to receive the parenting we missed earlier in our lives. God created us to be filled by Him *first* so

He may meet our deepest needs. The Bible promises God, as both Father and Mother, will meet every parental message listed.

1 John 4:8 declares, *"God is love."* We may not believe that God loves us, or that we're worthy of His love. That is a lie the enemy would have us believe. *God can't wait to lavish His love on you. He's crazy in love with you!* His most distinguishing character is His deep and endless love He has for every one of us; a love which satisfies completely.

† How does it make you feel to attach to your heavenly "mother"?

Daddy Holes

There's nothing in the world in a woman's heart like her daddy's love. And if you don't have your daddy's love, you'll look for it in all the wrong places, and sacrifice yourself to get it. —Iyanla Vanzant

He's my father!" I'd always say, defiantly, before running off to answer his calls or trying to see him while he was in town. Then like clockwork, in a few days or months, I'd be climbing back in mom's bed to lay my head on her lap, again. … He's disappointed me, again. That's what our relationship has always been, my father and me—an emotional roller coaster of irregular guest appearances. But still, I did not give up on him. *He's my father*—maybe I hoped saying those words over and over would somehow make them true. Even though I didn't know what having a father actually meant, I still wanted to have one—*mine*—anyway. … Perhaps there just wasn't room in his life to love all his children because he spent so much time chasing a high. I felt his absences. …

My relationship with my father taught me that no matter how much unconditional love you give to someone, getting love in return was not a guarantee. So, I found men who were distant charmers and loved me just as he did—selfishly. I attached myself to the smallest hint of affection, afraid of being left behind. … I felt abandoned and I couldn't shake that awful feeling that I should have been important enough for him to stay. –Danielle Rene, "Again"[77]

It's been said that a girl's father is the first man she loves. *There is nothing in the world like a daddy's love.* Today, sadly, many women have a "daddy hole" because Dad, or other significant male, such as a grandfather or stepfather, didn't or couldn't love his precious daughter the way she needed to be loved. (By the way, male abuse survivors quite often fear and avoid any affectionate contact with their own or other children.)

Girls need their dads in their lives for many reasons. There are certain things about life and relationships that only a father can teach his daughter. I now realize that despite my anger and frustration that my dad controlled so much of my life, negating my free will, I can say that he was always there for me.

Whatever our daddy hole, there's always hope for healing. The end of Danielle's story:

> We started communicating regularly through Facebook. I finally realized my dad is, like all of us, human. He's just a man, battling an addiction and years of his own hurts and bull. I now understand that his absences were likely an act of grace. Perhaps God spared me from the dark side of his life. ... I have *learned to forgive*, and I've come to a place of understanding what love is by *not* accepting what isn't. I've also stopped using my father's shortcomings as a reflection of my worth.[78]

To feel you're not important to a parent leaves you feeling "discarded," with a hole in your soul. Grieving and mourning the parent you never had is part of the healing process. Danielle came to the place where she faced reality. She grieved the father she never had and mourned the years stolen from her. Always remember: *Just because someone is unwilling or incapable of loving us, that doesn't mean we are unlovable.*

We might not have had a father who is around to help us and give us good fatherly advice, or who cares to truly know us, but we can call on our heavenly Father. He's never too busy to give us His full attention. God says He will be a father to the fatherless (Psalm 10:14; Genesis 21:8-20).

Take the mask off dad. When Jenna's dad was dying and she told him she loved him, he answered, "No one has ever loved me. No one ever wanted me." Instantly, her upbringing made total sense to Jenna.

† With Jesus, use this format to identify your Daddy losses.

Ways My Dad Let Me Down	*"Stuff" and Emotions I Struggle with Today*

Distorted Impressions of the Father

Whether you know it or not, your parents played an indirect role in your view of God, particularly your dad. When a healthy Dad is present, a child develops a more balanced view of God. This means that if your earthly dad didn't represent the character of God the Father, then God becomes guilty by association; He takes on your dad's characteristics.

God is a loving dad. That's what we hear in church. Yet, might you be one of those who when you hear "God is your father" you instinctively think of words like abandonment, loss, betrayal or unfaithfulness? Sadly, for centuries humans have had a totally false perception of God, a perception that threatened to destroy God's dream plan of sharing His joy and affection with His created.

Abuse usually magnifies our negative perceptions about God because at the heart of abuse is the misuse of power and control. And since God is *the* Power and Authority figure in the universe, He represents an abuse victim's greatest fears.

If mothers committed the abuse, the fatherhood of God can be problematic too. In these cases, survivors don't fear God will actively harm them, but they may believe He is passive: "If my earthly father didn't stop the abuse, then the heavenly Father won't be responsive either."

All distorted beliefs must be challenged.

I know God loves you more than you could possibly know. I know when you were being abused and wounded—so was God. God gives mankind free will, and man can be pretty evil and harming.

God *is* love (1 John 4:8) which means He cannot *not love*—He cannot not love you. You are His precious daughter. And He is a just God. Those who harmed you will be accountable to Him. It won't be pretty. He takes the health of your soul very seriously.

† What do you think is the hardest thing for you to experience in your relationship with God?

Over-Parenting

Perhaps you don't relate to this chapter's material. It certainly can help you develop empathy for those who have empty love tanks due to parental omissions. But there is another style of parenting, at the other end of the continuum, which can lead to difficulties in adulthood—"over-parenting," a.k.a. helicopter parenting, intensive parenting, bulldozing parenting, or s-mothering.

This parental style is mostly child-centered, emotionally absorbing, labor intensive, and doesn't nurture independence in children. It induces stress and anxiety, child experts agree. They tend to have emotional problems too.

A 2013 University of Mary Washington study found that college students who were raised by "helicopter" parents are more likely to be depressed. They also report less satisfaction with their lives overall; they have more health problems, and rely on medication.

These kids tend to grow up without learning how to regulate their emotions because their parents did that for them. If they were sad, their parents cheered them up. If they were mad, their parents calmed them down. Their lack of emotional regulation skills becomes a big problem once they leave the nest. Feeling entitled is a frequent mindset. Some parents may only over-parent one child, quite often the oldest or youngest, or a female. This leaves the other siblings feeling detached, unloved, and insignificant, thereby, creating a mommy and/or daddy hole.

Why are these parents so intense? Some recognize they never received good and healthy parental messages. Their desire is to give their kids what they didn't receive. Many harbor regrets about decisions they've made in their own lives; especially mothers. If moms believe they would have had better lives had they chosen differently when they were younger, they are more likely to be a helicopter parent. They usually have a mommy or daddy hole.

† Would you say you were over parented? If yes, what do you believe the consequences have been?

Technology

Although technology has improved our lives in profound ways, it has also presented a growing number of unique challenges.

Did you know it is really important to *look at your baby's face?* Not only do babies need hugs, to be talked to, tickled, diapered, and fed—*they need mom's constant eye contact.* This is how "emotional attachment style" or "bonding" is learned.

Today most moms have an obstacle that keeps them from making emotional eye contact and bonding effectively with their babies—their smartphone. What most moms don't know is they are retarding their baby's developmental window, which can lead to future impaired relationship attachments.[79]

Baby girls, in particular, are born interested in emotional expression. From these cues they discover whether they are worthy, lovable, or annoying. Take away an expressive face from a baby girl, and you take away the female brain's touchstone for realty, according to neuropsychiatrist, Louann Brizendine.

†††

I believe in most cases our parents parented us the best they could, given the emotional and physical resources they had. This is not about blame—it's about understanding our human condition; it's about why we think and do what we do; it's about recognizing we need to change our outcomes; about grieving the necessary losses and forgiveness—all so we can enjoy a better life and better connections. We can use this knowledge to become more protecting and mindful parents, grandparents, mentors, teachers or coaches.

6

HEALING FROM LOSS OF LOVE

It happened out of the blue. When I (Kimberly) didn't hear from him after an hour I started jumping to all kinds of conclusions. Three hours later, no word. I'm confused. The last thing I imagined is he'd be with someone else. After all, we'd been together for a number of idyllic years.

Bob was the man I loved with my entire heart and soul; the man I planned to spend rest of my life with. I spent that three-day holiday weekend alone, baffled, sick to my stomach, in shock, carrying a gut-wrenching pain that something had gone dreadfully wrong.

Nervous and fearful, I called him at work Tuesday morning and he was charming. He apologized and came over that night. It was an evening of reconciliation and ecstasy. He "teased" me into believing we were okay. He didn't have the backbone to break up with me, to tell me he'd found someone else. The next morning when he shut my front door, the only thing he left behind was a broken promise.

Two days later, as I was navigating my way through congested traffic, an intersection got jammed—and guess who was stuck right in front of me? Yep, Bob and "the other woman." Was this some kind of cruel joke? I stared straight into his face and he pretended not to see me. That's exactly how I felt—invisible. Like all the great memories had been erased by him.

It was a Cinderella moment. There on center stage stood the prince and his beautiful princess, as the ugly step-sister stood offstage, her heart completely ripped out.

Fury arose, *Liar! Jerk-off!* Then I just went cold. Trembling, I gathered what little dignity I had left and crawled into my office cubicle. I told a couple trustworthy co-workers what just happened.

Are you okay? I wouldn't feel okay for a very long time. I mean, how could he be so uncaring and just cut me off like that after so long?

The hardest truth to swallow was that my sadness had not been due to a death, but because someone I loved with my entire heart and soul, who I had bonded to willfully, chose to not be with me. Our intimate emotional and physical bond had been broken. I was knocked out twice. The first blow came when I realized he had sex with someone else; the second jolt came when I grasped that he'd been lying to me all along.

What's wrong with me? When I'd finally fall asleep, I'd wake up to the reality he was gone. Then my heart started re-bleeding. I couldn't muster up the energy to get out of bed and face the day.

By the way, when we first dated, I was "the other woman." He abandoned his girlfriend for me. As Dr. Phil says, "If they'll do it with you, they'll do it to you." I guess breaking up with him was like "dodging a bullet" as they say. But it didn't feel like that for me.

Betrayals often bring on posttraumatic stress and prompt an identity crisis. After Bob left, not only did I miss him and our lives together, but I missed feeling good about me. Any self-esteem I had, vanished. My bulimia spiraled out of control.

The shame of being "dumped" felt like I had a tattoo on my forehead: *Loser! Worthless!* No matter what I tried to do to feel better about myself, memories and nightmares of the desertion kept creeping up and drained any positive feelings I had about myself. The memories of abandonment and rejection affected my self-esteem for years due to lack of trust. The bottom line: I gave Bob too much power over my life.

We will all have loves in our lives that will let us go, and it stinks. Someone has chosen not to be with us; not to "keep us," to throw us away. In many cases the person chose to betray us. We will all have loves in our lives that will let us go, and it stinks. Someone has chosen not to be with us; not to "keep us."

Dancing in the Sonshine

In many cases the person chose to betray us. Some vulnerable women develop a *post-traumatic stress injury of abandonment* which can push them into a clinical depression, even suicide.

Sadly, there are "serial abandoners," those who get some reward from inflicting emotional pain on those who love them. For them, creating devastation is their way of exerting power over their mate. I was unfortunate enough to get engaged to one them! There's even a name for it: *Intimate Deception Betrayal Trauma (IDBT),* a form of post-traumatic stress (PTS). Perhaps we became the serial abandoner. The dynamics are no different than the abused woman who becomes an abuser. It's an act of self-protection and learned behavior.

Many factors affect how we react to the loss of a deep love: the nature and duration, the intensity of feelings, the circumstances of the breakup, our previous history of loss, our need to feel in control, and social support.

Depending upon the circumstances of the breakup, our personal history and physiology, we may develop a *post-traumatic stress injury of abandonment.* Severe stress caused by loss of relationship can push the vulnerable into a clinical depression, even suicide.

Why such devastating results? When we were born, we were programmed to love and be loved. It's not only intimate partner relationships. We also know that child neglect, abandonment and abuse are a horrible kind of betrayal. Parents are among the most potent and significant influences in our lives. Someone tricked or took advantage of an established, trusting, loving relationship.

The content in this chapter can be applied to any close and warm relationships. And let us never forget that there is One who will never let us go. *"I'm in a desperate situation!" David replied to Gad. "But let me fall into the hands of the LORD, for his mercy is very great"* (1 Chronicles 21:13)

† In ways do you relate to my story and this material?

The Physiological Pain

You are lovable even if the most important person in your world rejects you, you are still real, and you are still okay. —Melody Beattie, Codependent No More

The wounds of abandonment and healing process is immensely complex because part of us dies. There's often no satisfying closure. When a life partner betrays us, we are afflicted by the person we chose as one of the most powerful influences in our life.

To find evidence that one's mate is having an affair may be the most awful pain a person can ever experience. The same can be said for a parent choosing to desert their child.

"Abandonment." It's about loss of love and connectedness, an incident that suddenly happens, or after a period of months, perhaps years. It's an *involuntary separation on the part of one partner.*

Abandonment isn't like an accident from which we begin to immediately heal. It's more like spending weeks or months on a battlefield, constantly under attack. Each time we think about it, the brain triggers the release of stress hormones, which is why people become ill; barely able to function.

Whenever a breakup takes place there is disappointment, confusion, and pain because a tight bond has been broken.[80] *Rejection* is one of our most powerful emotions. It is a threat to our identity; to the entire self. It can cause as much distress in the pain center of the brain as an actual physical injury, according to research. The brain actually feels the pain of neurochemical withdrawal, similar to a drug withdrawal state. Without love's regular surges of the hormone *dopamine*, a depression-despair response kicks in.[81]

Physically, the body reacts as if our heart had literally been stabbed or punched in the gut.[82] There's a reason. It's been said that humans have two brains: one in the gut (the gut is our GI tract: esophagus, stomach and intestines) and the one sitting in our skull. These two brains are in direct communication with each other through the hefty *vagus nerve.* This gut-brain connection can link anxiety to stomach problems and vice versa. Have you ever had a "gut-wrenching" experience? No wonder experts say to listen to our gut! Add to this that women's brains are marinated in *estrogen*. We're hard-wired for connection. When a relationship falls apart, the normal sadness a person would feel affects more neurons an area *eight times larger* in the female brain than in the male brain.[83]

Have you noticed women will fight harder to save a relationship than a guy? Males are trained to "cut their losses." For females, a loss of relationship triggers a hormonal change that strengthens the feelings of abandonment or loss. "A woman feels more deeply" has an actual physiological basis.[84] Motivation for a reunion is high because the hormonal rush of *oxytocin* and *dopamine* suppresses anxiety and disbelief, reinforcing love circuits in the brain.

† Describe what thoughts and feeling have risen in you.

We Don't Want to See It

In my life, I bore four incredibly painful breakups. Each guy decided to discard me like a piece of garbage. And what I learned is that *people can't give you what they don't have*. If he doesn't have empathy, I won't receive empathy. If he's not honest, he can't give me honesty. If he's never experienced a healthy relationship or unconditional love, he can't give me that. I'll be waiting forever for change to happen … unless he recognizes he needs help and pursues changing. The fact that someone chose not to be with me says more about that person and the condition of the relationship.

I have to admit that *I didn't want to see; I didn't want to know*. Unawareness (denial) is a powerful survival technique. We remain blind to betrayal and the signs in order to protect ourselves. When the rose-colored glasses of healing were removed, I realized my relationships failed because they were built on the physical, not on the emotional and spiritual. And I was co-dependent.

Without help and God, many people never completely recover from the loss of love. True restoration means confronting uncomfortable feelings, understanding what they are, and more importantly, learning how to grieve them—with God.

No matter how upsetting or demoralizing the circumstances may have been, *you are not undeserving of love.* Believe it or not, Jesus felt the pain of betrayal too. His friends abandoned Him in the last hours, and then on the cross. He cried out asking why His own Father had turned away.

Be assured that Jesus understands how you feel since He experienced abandonment Himself. You can talk to Him about your memories and feelings and heartaches.

† In what ways do you relate?

The Stages and Emotions We Traverse

Not belonging is a terrible feeling. It feels awkward and it hurts, as if you were wearing someone else's shoes. —Phoebe Stone, The Romeo and Juliet Code

Every person is wired for love differently, yet according to experts, most people follow a predictable pattern proceeding a distressing break-up or abandonment.

Stage 1—*Shattering:* a bond of human attachment broken; a feeling of devastation and unbearable pain; shock, panic, suddenly void of life's worth and meaning. There's a big difference between being *broken* and being *shattered.* Think of a vase. If the vase breaks, you can put it back together with super glue. If it's shattered, it's destroyed. That's what being "shattered" feels like, doesn't it?

Stage 2—*Intense love withdrawal,* which has been compared to heroin withdrawal. This stage lasts the longest and is the most intense stage. Emotions vacillate. We experience a powerful craving and unrest for the love we're missing. We wait for our beloved to return; to come to their senses—all because we're wired by God for attachment.

For reasons of emotional survival, injured people attempt to find ways to control the damage following the injury. One way is to hang onto love, and suppress the anger and the truth, so we can hang onto hope. We often try to find a way to cope via a coping or defense mechanism, whether with food, drugs, work, sex, shopping, social media, TV, overcleaning, gambling, romance novels or movies—all of which are intended to help us escape instead of addressing our problem head-on.

There's something wrong with them! We make a vow to our heart, *That's the last time I'll let anyone shake me like that again.* We think we're protecting ourselves, but in reality, we're only trapping ourselves in a pattern of behavior that binds us to bitterness and depression.

Rage is a coping mechanism which may surface. It's our way of protesting against the pain and fighting back; an unconscious refusal to be victimized by someone leaving us. We may unconsciously create *contempt for men*. We may find ourselves blaming some guy in the present for something this betrayer did to us in the past.

Some women make demands, begging him to come back, promising to change. They may become ill or more dependent, act out, or attempt suicide. To her, this is the only form of control she has in the aftermath of a devastating injury.

Shame is common. *There's something inherently wrong with me if I can't hold onto this guy. How could I, a smart lady, not see this coming? How could I have let this happen?* At the heart of shame is the belief that we're undeserving of love, which is a dangerous belief.

Stage 3—*Internalize the rejection.* "Internalizing" means making it part of yourself. Old wounds tend to open back up, spilling their toxins into the new sore creating a bigger wound. All the past rejections merge with the present one, creating a new toxic memory.

We turn on ourselves. *If only I had …* We become preoccupied with regrets over the relationship, agonizing over what *should have* or *could have* been done to prevent the traumatic outcome. This only leaves us feeling more worthless and hopeless.

Yet, along with the rage, shame, blame, hate, sorrow, guilt and pain, we still feel love, at least until we can sort it all out. If we choose to let go of the love, we know we'll have to feel the full force of the injury. Who wants that? As we hang onto the love, we hang onto whatever control we have left.

It's easy to get stuck in either or both stages 2 and 3 because of lack of closure.

Stage 4—*Acceptance.* Someone once said, "You've got to learn to leave the table when love's no longer being served." When we realize we weren't able to control what happened, nor able to restore the relationship, and the relationship has ended, reality sets in. Accepting loss is a slow and painful process because often there is little or no sufficient closure. Yet, God can provide the closure we need.

Stage 5—*Mourn.* Although it takes two people to form an intimate relationship, it only takes one to end it. With God by our side, the day comes when we accept the reality of the loss, grieve it, and move forward. We need to grieve the numerous losses associated with the relationship (not find a "rebound" guy). For example, we may have grown close to his family and his circle of friends = additional loss.

Stage 6—*Hope* is the final stage. God is ready to lift us up and out of the anguish and into a purpose-driven life; to help us restructure life and let go of the pain. He always has a better ending.

† How well do you relate to these stages? If you are struggling in one of these stages, what is Hope saying to you?

Wired for Love

We all have a hole in our heart that longs for completeness, so the illusion of perfect romantic love is appealing. At age 30, I decided to venture out and meet men by shopping the newspaper classified "Personals." Today it would be *Match.com* or *eHarmony* or one of a hundred dating sites available online. It was my way to gain control and choose my own "perfect man."

I was so desperate for a deep, loving connection that I answered over 100 personal ads (and a hilarious manuscript came out of it). However, after about the 50th date, I realized what you read is not what you get.

In the movie *Sleepless in Seattle,* Rosie O'Donnell's character says, "You don't want to be in love; you want to be in love with a movie." That was me! In my defense, seeking a potential mate is how God designed me.

Let's look a little deeper at why our love relationships go awry by looking into the female brain. (Reference: New York Times bestseller, *The Female Brain,* by Dr. Louanne Brizendine.) Once we understand how we're wired by God, then we can let go of any guilt and shame we've attached to a broken relationship. Our challenge is to build a new life and new healthy relationships, whether it be a romantic companion, a friendship, or enhancing family connections.

Let's look at my situation: I agree to meet Aron, whom I've just met on the telephone (I answered his personal ad). We agree to meet at a local bar and restaurant. Walking in, all of my attention circuits will be on "mating alert status." If Aron, or for that matter any prospective guy, makes eye contact with me, I immediately wonder about his relationship status. *Is he single or hiding the fact he's married?*

My attention is riveted on his face and physique, comparing it to what's in my mind's photo album of guys who attract and seduce me (these images are hardwired into our brain's "love drive").

As Aron greets me, my brain begins to imprint everything about him. I'm initially attracted to him so my hormones surge. I begin calculating the qualities that might put him in the running as a potential mate. Waves of attraction and desire flood my body with a rush of *dopamine,* sparking euphoria and excitement. My brain shoots out some *testosterone,* the hormone that stokes sexual desire. It's a "woo-hoo" encounter.

Aron is handsome, funny, charming, and "appears" to have his life together. But I need to be sure on a gut level I can trust him. So, my brain starts to calculate if there's any potential danger. A natural cautiousness towards strangers is part of the brain's wiring—unless you're intoxicated, like I usually was. Therefore, I didn't connect with my natural fear circuits, so I put myself into high-risk situations.

With a "sober" female, due to this extra cautiousness, her brain isn't ready to admit being over-infatuated or excited about sex as compared to a male. If she has a mommy or daddy hole (a depleted love tank) and craves a parent's embrace, she may easily throw caution to the wind, as I did.

Then I wonder, *Do you think I'm okay—pretty? Do you accept me?* If he appears to answer yes, then I think, *Love me! Let's become inseparable!* The act of hugging or cuddling releases *oxytocin* in the brain and produces a tendency to trust the "hugger." It also increases the likelihood that you'll believe everything and anything he tells you.

Our thinking succumbs to "wishful thinking." We convince ourselves, at least for a while, that he's "the one," that there is truth in everything he has said. Our friends may alert us to some red flag but we cherry-pick the evidence (denial). If he tells us he "loves" us and our best friend has seen him with another woman, we won't believe he is being unfaithful. *It's his sister or his neighbor!*

The tendency is to cling to our beliefs, even in the face of contradicting evidence (which applies to all aspects of our lives). Studies have shown that we tend to slant the way we process information in such a way as to preserve our underlying and false beliefs.[85] If things aren't so great, human beings will deceive themselves to make things look rosier. We deal with reality by unconsciously distorting it—and those distortions can serve as a protective function by insulating us from harm.

Meeting an Abuser for the First Time

Let's assume the guy you meet is an abuser. Nothing changes as far as your mind and body is concerned, but an abuser thinks differently than most men. According to abuse expert Don Hennessey,

Before the (skilled) abuser initiates contact with a prospective long-term partner, he has already developed some very strong beliefs and attitudes. In his own mind, he knows what he needs from an intimate relationship and he is convinced that he is entitled to have these needs met. He's also convinced these needs outweigh any cost to his prospective partner. He believes he's entitled to be the center of any adult relationship.

With his beliefs and attitudes well developed, he will initiate a contact where he can assess the possibility of acting out his agenda. The meeting is designed to allow him to check out the possibility of beginning a relationship where he'll be in charge. He'll do this without her being aware she is being targeted. Right from the first encounter he is listening to and evaluating everything she reveals. She will be unaware she is being invited to develop a relationship where her wishes will be suppressed, and where the wishes of him become paramount. This invitation is enveloped in whatever language the abuser believes will work. He will present a story about himself that will inevitably lead her to being more attracted to him.

Undoubtably, the tactics of abuse and control are hidden from the woman. If his assessment is that the woman is incapable or unwilling to put him first and follow his wishes, he may move on to another target.[86]

† Explain why you do or do not relate to this material?

The In-Love Addicted Brain

You are addicted to love because you are made in God's image (God is love).
—Caroline Leaf, PhD, The Perfect You

Aron and I hit it off and had a couple of dates. I started to feel "in love." You're probably not surprised to learn that the brain becomes "illogical" when it comes to romance; literally blind to the beloved's shortcomings.

Once a person falls "in love," the cautious, critical-thinking pathways in the brain shut down. We're less likely to see any red flags because our beloved's faults don't matter, hence the term, "Love is blind." It's an involuntary state because the frenzied brain is running on the neurochemicals: *dopamine, estrogen, oxytocin,* and *testosterone.*

Meryl, an intelligent woman and mother of four, is separated from her abusive husband. In counseling, she'd describe the horrible things he did one minute but would then come up with a reason to call him. She'd do this despite the very fact he was dangerous.

"I think I'm obsessed with this man. Yes, that's it, he's my addiction!" Meryl claimed she couldn't figure it out. She didn't feel loving toward him. She didn't respect nor trust him. She couldn't understand why she had this desire to stay involved with him.

The brain circuits that are activated when we feel "in love" match those of the drug addict desperately craving the next fix. In the *Psychology Today* online article "Can Love Be an Addiction?" Lori Jean Glass, revealed she was diagnosed with an addiction to being in love, also called "partner addiction." For her, the addiction involved being completely absorbed in someone else's life, and the feeling that someone else needed her and admired her. Someone, anyone; it didn't matter who it was as long as it was a warm body capable of overflowing her brain with love chemicals.

Robert Palmer's 1988 song "You're going to have to face it, you're addicted to love" is sickeningly familiar. Numerous studies have found the same brain neurochemicals are in play as with drug addiction (massive amounts of *serotonin, dopamine,* and *norepinephrine*). They both activate the same reward pathways in the brain. The brain's fear-alert system, and its worrying and critical thinking system, are turned way down when the love circuits are running on full blast, much the same when people are taking Ecstasy. Romantic love is a natural Ecstasy high.

From the brain's perspective, whatever we do to produce feelings of euphoria, is worth repeating. Maybe we've mastered our addiction to food, or work, or a substance. Now we find we're obsessed with our beloved. Love addiction is just as real as any other addiction in terms of its behavior patterns and brain mechanisms. And *withdrawal,* as in ending the relationship, can be extremely painful, just like substance addiction.

† † †

Many of us need to change the way we're doing relationships. We need to take a "time-out" to allow God to show us how to change our thinking and behavior to get a better result. Sometimes we need to take time away from relationship drama to see the mistakes we've made and to see God's perspective.

In order to really love someone, we have to know them well; we have to spend hours just talking because there's so much to learn. Many of us are terrified of being intimately known. We know the ugly parts of our souls. We're afraid it's only a matter of time before the truth surfaces and we're rejected once again. Real love is like God—pure, just, and perfect. This is why it's so important to understand love from God's point of view.

† I believe you should avoid a new love relationship for *at least* 6-months; one year is ideal. *Taking time to heal emotionally is a critical part of helping you move on and choose a healthy partner.* In what ways do you agree or disagree?

Today's Pain—Yesterday's Abandonment

Every fool can see what is wrong. See what is good in it! –Winston Churchill

Patrice summarized a recent date she had, "I only had *one date* with this guy. He didn't call me the next day like he said he would. I'm totally stressed about this. I was sure he really liked me. I can't believe I'm this upset over just one date with a guy I really don't even know!" Then Patrice had a revelation and asked, "Could my feelings be unresolved grief over past relationships that went sour?"

Yes. Being left by someone we love can open up old wounds, stir insecurities and doubts, going all the way back to childhood. A relationship that ended today may be for you the fulfillment of your worst nightmares from childhood—the fear of being left alone and abandoned like you were by a caregiver or significant person.

Or, if you find yourself asking: *Why can't I make this work? Why aren't I lovable? Why can't I get him to love me back?* —it all may be rooted in the lingering insecurity and fear stemming from long-lost loves.

Imprinted in the brain (*amygdala*) are memories of how we've responded to fear and other perceived threats since infancy. The amygdala continues to gather emotional memories as we grow. Once it has been conditioned to an emotional response, such as feeling anxious when a loved one threatens separation, the memory slate never gets completely wiped clean, so to speak. Emotions and sensations reminiscent of the original abandonment memory activate the amygdala's circuits, and you once again experience the emotions and needs from that earlier loss, all over again.

As a kid, Keaton's father berated her for every mistake and fault. Consequently, Keaton felt rejected and blamed herself for not being good enough. As a teen, she could never shake the feeling that she needed to prove herself. She was extremely sensitive to peer rejection. When her first boyfriend broke up with her at age 17, she became depressed and started experimenting with marijuana. This romantic rejection confirmed old feelings of inadequacy.

Going into adulthood, what followed was a chain of short-lived and volatile relationships gone bad. Whenever Keaton became overcome with romantic pain, she drowned her feelings in alcohol. With every breakup she said she felt like a relationship failure, like she had a disease. She lost all hope of ever finding real love.

Add to this peer rejection. When I (Kimberly) was in 2nd grade, our family moved from America to England. Nothing was normal anymore. On the first day of school I attended my first gym class. Unbeknownst to our family, the boys and girls had gym together. Each child was dressed in uniform underwear—dark navy-blue "knickers" (English for panties) and a thick, stark white undershirt.

I slithered into the gym wearing a flimsy undershirt with a cute little bow and worn out, flowery underpants with a big hole along the elastic line! The kids laughed and pointed at me. *Weird kid from America.* No one wanted me in their group or on their team, leaving me devastated. This memory was imprinted and activated each time I was rejected by a guy, particularly during my school years.

Wanted by the Father

Truth be told, someone has always wanted me—a lot—my heavenly Father.

- Hosea 11:8: *Oh, how can I give you up, Israel* [my beloved children]*? How can I let you go? ... My heart is torn within me, and my compassion overflows.*
- Zephaniah 3:17*: The LORD your God will take great delight in you, he will quiet you with his love, he will rejoice over you with singing.*
- Jeremiah 31:3*: I* [God] *have loved you with an everlasting love; I have drawn you with loving-kindness.*

Pursue the One Who Is Pursuing You
As I meditate on and believe God's Word about me, I can stop looking at myself and seeing what is wrong. I'm the fool. Pastor Bob Sorge wrote,

> Until you are established on the inside in the love of God, you will always be susceptible to rejection's wounding. Those who have not learned to find their satisfaction in the Father's acceptance always end up looking for it in all the wrong places. And instead of finding the acceptance they long for, they get rejected all over again. The only place of everlasting acceptance is in the arms of your loving Savior.[87]

God Will Never Abandon You—

- Deuteronomy 31:6*: Be strong and courageous. Do not be afraid or terrified because of them, for the LORD your God goes with you; he will never leave you nor forsake you* [give up on you]*.*

- Isaiah 62:4: *No longer will they call you Deserted, or name your land Desolate. But you will be called Hephzibah, and your land Beulah; for the LORD will take delight in you.*

God Heals—

- Psalm 147:3 *God heals the brokenhearted and binds up their wounds.*
- Revelation 21:4: *He will wipe every tear from their eyes. There will be no more death or mourning or crying or pain …*

† I challenge you to meditate and hold your thoughts for at least 12 minutes on these Scriptures each day. Ponder what each word means and what God is saying to you and about you. In a matter of weeks, you'll begin to build and strengthen your relationship with God—and new neural circuits in your brain of compassion and empathy!

Love Yourself the Way God Does

We're "abandonment survivors"—those who have lost and loved and experienced the anguish. It is not uncommon to fear loving again. Love is one of the most captivating powers we possess as human beings. We may not be able to control the love of another, but we can increase our own capacity to give and receive love. It begins with allowing God to heal our abandonment wounds with His power and love, then learning to love ourselves. Until we can love ourselves as God does, we will have a tough time loving another person and accepting someone else's authentic love.

Remember the love tank analogy. If our love tank isn't full, we don't have the right kind of love to give another person or receive from another person. It all begins with loving ourselves properly.

Alanna always wondered, *Why is it so hard to love myself?* It's been said that we tend to treat ourselves as we've been treated. If you've been in a relationship with a person who has abandoned, or controlled, or devalued you, then you probably don't think about your own needs. You only think about what is wrong with you.

Loving, having compassion, accepting the goodness, and valuing yourself is the beginning of making your life better. Many of us are familiar with 1 Corinthians 13, dubbed, "God's Love Chapter."

Did you know there are over 1000 ideas for the use of this Scripture on Pinterest? Most sermons on this passage revolve around the teaching of Christian love for God and others. Yet, verses 4-9 illustrate not only how we are to love God and one another, but how we can truly love ourselves. This may be the first time you learn to love yourself. The more we understand who God made us to be, the more skilled we will be at distinguishing between acting on impulse and listening to the Spirit's nurturing voice inside us.

> *Love is patient, love is kind. It does not envy, it does not boast, it is not proud. It does not dishonor others, it is not self-seeking, it is not easily angered, and it keeps no record of wrongs. Love does not delight in evil but rejoices with the truth. It always protects, always trusts, always hopes, always perseveres. Love never fails.*

When Paul wrote this, he had in mind a character sketch of Christ. He is thinking of a Jesus-kind-of-patience; a Jesus-kind-of-kindness; etc., which Jesus imparts into our souls, making living out these qualities possible.

- *Love is patient.* Often, we're more patient with other people (the people who hurt us) than we are with ourselves. Be less hard and more tolerant with yourself.
- *Love is kind.* Treating ourselves kindly is to protect and take proper care of our bodies, minds and spirits; and whatever else God has given us charge over (such as children, a job, education, ministry). Give yourself permission to be gentle and caring to yourself.
- *Love does not envy or boast; is not proud.* Many of us have created carefully constructed masks to hide our perceived inadequacies and grief—masks that brag, boast, gossip or display jealousy. Taking off our masks and seeing ourselves as God sees us, reveals our God-created selves—humble, empathetic and gentle.

- *Love keeps no records of wrongs.* Forgive yourself when you mess up. Because you've been forgiven by God this means getting rid of guilty and shame-based feelings; all records of wrongs.
- *Love rejoices in the truth.* You may have been told you're a loser, or fat and ugly; that you're unwanted and insignificant. God, your Creator and Papa, never said these things. He said you are a saint, and holy and precious!
- *Love trusts.* We can rest assure that if we're in God's will and following His instructions, then our choices will be trustworthy.
- *Love always hopes.* Oswald Chambers wrote, "Every hope and dream of the human mind will be fulfilled if it is noble and of God." Focus continually on God and believe in a bright future.
- *Love protects.* We're responsible to stay safe, protect ourselves and our children. We don't have control over another person's actions, but we can control how we prepare and respond to circumstances.
- *Love perseveres.* Don't give up on yourself. Everyday God gives you a new source of strength and power! Use it!
- *Love never fails.* We must believe and move forward knowing God will always be there and has a great plan for our lives (Jeremiah 29:11). He always completes what He begins (Romans 8:29). I love what Lisa Bevere wrote, "If you think you've blown God's plan for your life, rest in this: you are not that powerful."

† Finish these sentences:

- What is right about me (what I celebrate with God about me) is …
- I add value to this world by …

Get Support

In this culture it is easy to underestimate our human need for connection. We live separated, in relative isolation from one another, even family. To begin healing from abandonment issues, we need to become reliant on God and other people. First, we should always be over-reliant on God. Second, we need friends, family, pastors, and professionals for nurturance.

Support from others. When my guys left me, I realized just how dependent I had become on them (codependent). I didn't have any best friends I could go to for support. I had to learn to cultivate new friendships.

Researchers found that people who have been exposed to crises find that social support and relationships with others are key predictors of psychological, physical, and spiritual restoration. The primary protective factor against developing PTSD is having relationships that provide care, support, love, trust, and encouragement.

How often do we cry out to Jesus in the face of tragedy and injustice, "Jesus, why don't You do something?" Too often we don't hear His response: *I am doing something—through the Church; through the people who belong to Me!* Look at the people around you who strengthen, stand with and encourage you. See God in them.

Someone said, "It doesn't matter who hurt you, or broke you down. What matters is who made you smile again." We need help from our sisters-in-Christ to mourn our losses.

Lana said, "I'm glad we're talking about this. I feel calmer just acknowledging I don't like it, and I'm in the company of others who also don't like it." It's important to surround ourselves with people who can simply hear us. The Bible tells us to,

- *"Pray for each other so that you may be healed. The prayer of a righteous man is powerful and effective" (James 5:16).*
- *"Rejoice with those who rejoice, weep with those who weep" (Romans 12:15);*
- *"Therefore encourage one another and build one another up, just as you are doing" (1 Thessalonians 5:11).*

7

THE WAY OF TRANSITION

Aimee, a lawyer at a top Manhattan firm, has "everything." Cindy has a list of extraordinary accomplishments. Darlene's busy lifestyle and powerful ministry attract admiration. Despite their impressive exteriors, these women feel completely empty inside. Aimee lost her virginity when a school mate raped her; Cindy's self-confidence vanished when her mother repeatedly told her she was stupid, ugly and wished she'd never been born. Darlene lost her husband and home when she divorced. These women experienced huge losses. And for each big loss suffered, they each experienced numerous *secondary losses*.

Abuse is a personal invasion and cause for deep grief. What we're going to see now is there is a profound connection between post-traumatic stress/PTSD and loss and grief. Abused women (and children) experience countless intangible losses, which society rarely recognizes as grief. For example,

- Loss of our health (chronic illness or injury; addiction).
- Loss of ability to or choice to have children (infertility; a failed adoption; abortion; a career or person took priority).
- Loss of normalcy and freedom (being forced to endure and cope with things that make no sense at all).
- Loss of—trust, safety, childhood or a stage of life.
- Loss of love.
- Loss of a parent's love (nurture) or presence (divorce; abandonment).
- Loss of memory ("Where was my childhood. I don't have any memories.")
- Loss of a home, husband and/or children.
- Loss of self—of intimacy, of control over our bodies and minds.

- Loss for the girl who wasn't allowed to have feelings.
- Loss of something we never had (like a healthy intimate relationship with other family members).
- Loss of healthy socialization; of value and respect for ourselves.
- Loss of joy, peace, and happiness.
- Loss of expectations and dreams; career opportunities.

Have you felt confused as to why you may always feel "down" or sad? It may be because your mind and heart are grieving many losses. Greif isn't just about feeling sad. The mind can become consumed with *shock, denial, exploding emotions, numbness, disbelief, confusion, anger, fear, regret, panic, guilt,* and *depression* as it struggles with accepting reality.

A divorce, for example, is trauma. It's a crisis which can become chronic—emotionally, physically and spiritually. When a couple breaks up, it means not only grieving the present losses, but the future the couple dreamed of. These losses are reasons to feel anguish and sadness. They quite often take a toll on the body.

Grief and heartache are natural responses to an injury and its successive losses. So, *losses, both intangible and tangible, need to be recognized and then mourned* so we can begin to rebuild a sense of self, trust and safety.

† When you read this list of losses, do you see some areas of your life that you may never have considered as a loss? Explain.

Good Grief

Grief is about strong emotional feelings caused by the end of, or change in, the familiar. It is not the same for everyone and there doesn't appear to be specific stages a person must go through. Symptoms can be mild, extreme, or somewhere in between.

Grief isn't always about death; it happens in relationships. We can say people in abusive relationships *experience death*—a gradual slow, confusing, and painful psychological death; some do physically die.

Have you noticed in this society we're given permission to grieve a person's death, but other losses like divorce or leaving an abusive marriage go unrecognized or are minimized? When a loved one dies, friends and family bring food and send sympathy cards. When a relationship ends due to abuse, the victim is often judged for ending the marriage, "She chose to leave." Friends and family may applaud you for getting out, but rarely do they console you because they don't understand the pain and despair.

In other words, we're expected to swallow the pain. No one brings casseroles or sends sympathy cards. Let me add, that grieving is not necessarily tied to leaving or ending a relationship. We can do a lot of grieving while still in an abusive relationship.

What if Post-Traumatic Stress (PTS) is really a form of grief? If you think about it, PTS is really a form of grief because when we experience a traumatic event—a personal injury—we experience profound losses.[88] Dr. Alan Wolfelt has done extensive work with both PTS and grieving patients. He calls PTS "traumatic grief."[89] Therefore, we can say: *PTSD is grief* set in motion by a traumatic event.

Everything you've been doing so far has been preparing you for the grief process and to transition you to post-traumatic growth. I call this chapter "the hinge" of the study. If this chapter were deleted, the key to understanding pain and healing would have no meaning.

My challenge is how to best present an unpleasant reality called grief, so you can confront it and be changed by it. I trust God to walk you through this process. As one psychologist put it, "Denying grief work doesn't work well in the long run."

Dr. James Pennebaker at the University of Texas discovered that keeping our experiences locked away inside us, never discussed, can do even more harm, and may even be more damaging than the actual traumatic event.

Dr. Alan Wolfelt wrote, "We cannot skirt the outside edges of our grief. Instead, we must journey all through it, sometimes meandering the side roads, sometimes plowing directly into its raw center. We must experience it, then we must express it."

† How *confident* would you say you feel about doing the grief work?

1	2	3	4	5	6	7	8	9	10
Not confident									Extremely confident

To Transition is to Express Grief

There is a difference between loss, grief and mourning:

- *Loss* is an *outcome* of an event or experience. For example, a divorce.
- *Grief* is the total of everything we think and feel *inside* after experiencing that loss; an *inward* heart-felt emotion. *I feel depressed. I feel numb. I feel so sad. I'm bitter and resentful. I feel powerless.*
- *Mourning* is the *outward* expression of grief. *I'm sad for the things I lost, and what I'll never have or be. Who might I be now if I hadn't been abused? I cry. I talk about what happened. I work through recovery exercises.*

Mourning is the active part of the PTSI healing journey—it's our medicine. There are wonderful treatment plans out there for PTSD like EMDR *(Eye Movement Desensitization and Reprocessing)* and specific cognitive behavioral therapies. But let's say we only focus on only eliminating PTSD symptoms and exclude the grief process and ignore the internal heart break—this is like having a triple-bypass surgery without changing your diet or exercise habits. The surgery can fix the immediate, life-threatening symptoms, but unless it's followed by a holistic self-care plan, overall health and well-being won't likely improve. The same can be said for PTSD treatment that doesn't focus on the traumatic grief and mourning.

This can be hard, but if we don't mourn then we may experience symptoms of *complicated grief*. What happens is when we're in a long-term abusive relationship, we accumulate losses year after year, then we feel overwhelmed by all the losses. Our pain gets stuck or off-track, and we find it hard to return to normal activities; to life.

Leaving Scrooge Behind

In Charles Dickens' classic *A Christmas Carol,* we meet the miserly Scrooge who is visited by three ghosts. The ghost of Christmas past takes Scrooge to his childhood where he recalls a series of unhappy moments: his father abandons him at a boarding school; his young sister dies; he rejects his fiancé in order to make more money. The ghost of Christmas present shows Scrooge the kindness of his employee's family (the Cratchits), whose smallest member, Tiny Tim, is dying—a direct result of Scrooge's refusal to pay Bob Cratchit a decent wage. When the spirit of Christmas future shows Scrooge his own neglected state, Scrooge is at last transformed.

Scrooge doesn't change because he's frightened—he changes because he's haunted, which is the same as saying he was 'convicted' by the Holy Spirit. Conviction alerts us to some truthful fact that we're trying to avoid. What was Scrooge trying to avoid? It turns out that he didn't want to think about the death of his mother and sister, or the loss of his fiancé. He couldn't bear the thought that love ends. Scrooge changes because the ghosts uncover his delusion that you can live a life without loss. They undo his delusion by haunting Scrooge with the losses he has already experienced, and the inevitable loss of what's going on around him.

Scrooge can't redo his past, nor can he really be certain of the future. Waking up on Christmas morning, thinking in a new way, he can change his present. This is important because living stuck in the past, and/or avoiding our feelings of loss sand sadness, can only leave us feeling helpless and depressed.

What we see in *A Christmas Carol* is that when Scrooge grieves for those he loved; he comes to life!

What we are talking about is a way of *transitioning;* coming to terms with a "new normal." Just like grief, transitions in life have a way of dropping on us unexpectedly. A common example is the difficult time a couple has dealing with the loss of time and freedom that comes with having a newborn baby. Before they can enjoy their miracle child, they have to deal with the ending of their old life of freedom.

Before we can fully enjoy the restored life God has for us, we may have to deal with the ending of our old life (and old coping mechanisms). Second Corinthians 5:17 states, *"Therefore if anyone is in Christ, she is a new creature; the **old things passed away**; behold, new things have come."*

To enjoy a new beginning, we need to acknowledge an ending. The Bible tells us there is a time to tear down and build (transition) and a time mourn (Eccl. 3:3-4). God is all about walking us through this. He reminds us that our pain is not our identity, that as surely as we pass through the painful emotions, we'll in time come out of the dark valley into the light.

> *God will "comfort all who mourn and provide for those who grieve—He'll give them a crown of beauty instead of ashes, the oil of joy instead of mourning, and a garment of praise instead of a spirit of despair (Isaiah 61:2).*

The objective is to *face the loss* and *work on adapting to it, and finally accept it*. The good news is: For most of us, grief is not overwhelming or unending. Although seemingly unbearable at times, it causes us to grow in ways that might not be possible otherwise.

Dr. George Bonanno, a specialist in bereavement and author of *The Other Side of Sadness,* wrote,

> Grief, above all, is a human experience. It is something we are wired for and it is certainly not meant to overwhelm us. ... I am amazed by how resilient humans are, and I have been working with loss and trauma survivors for years. ... The struggle may last anywhere from a few hours to a few days to a few weeks, sometimes longer, but most of us find a way to regain equilibrium and get on with our lives.[90]

It is important to listen to the inner gentle whisper of the Holy Spirit. If we are willing, He will show you what truths and losses you haven't acknowledge, and what work needs to be done.

† Just because a loss, such as giving up a reliable yet destructive coping mechanism, is unhealthy, it doesn't mean we do not need to mourn this loss—this "old thing." How does this feel to do?

The Mourning Tool Box

Here are your two primary "power tools" to help you transform pain to sadness; grief and loss to God-joy.

Prayer

Luke 6:12 tells us, *"Now it came to pass in those days that [Jesus] went out to the mountain to pray, and continued all night in prayer to God."*

If Jesus, the Son of God, needed to go to His Father in prayer for strengthening and guidance, how much more do we (Psalm 32:6)? Yet, have you ever felt that your heart and mind are so on overload that you cannot pray?

When we're diagnosed with cancer, or lose a job or a friendship ends, the force of the storm threatens our prayer life because in those moments we're not able to see how we'll ever keep from breaking completely apart.

God understands. In fact, He understands so much the Spirit will actually pray for us. The Message version of Romans 8:26 tells us,

> *The moment we get tired in the waiting, God's Spirit is right alongside helping us along. If we don't know how or what to pray, it doesn't matter. He does our praying in and for us, making prayer out of our wordless sighs, our aching groans.*

For the most part, we are able to pray. And it's the first thing we should do when our soul is in conflict. Prayer is talking honestly to God—at any time; in any place. Philippians 4:6 says to *"pray about everything."* Nothing is too trivial for Him to listen to.

Prayer is anticipating God's faithfulness; it's having the faith each prayer has been accepted and heard and received by God.

Matthew 20:32 reads, *"Jesus stopped and called, "What do you want me to do for you?"* He's asking you the same thing. Be specific with your request.

Schedule a Prayerful Grief Appointment

When Jesus heard that his cousin, John the Baptist, had been beheaded, *"he left in a boat to a remote area to be alone" (Matthew 14:13)*. In addition to a group of safe people, we need to deal with our grief alone, as Jesus did. Yet Jesus didn't dwell on His pain endlessly; He returned to His ministry. We can follow His example.

In order to avoid getting flooded by emotions day in and day out, many counselors (including me) suggest "scheduling" processing our emotions by creating a specific time to meet with God in order to grieve the pain and loss—*a prayerful grief appointment*. This would also be the time you would journal your emotions. It may also be a time when you work through a recovery book.

Think of it as putting a boundary or a fence around your emotions. Then when you're done for the day, you go back to what's going on in the present world. One method that works is to commit to a 14 to 30-day period. Each day, or every other day, set your timer for anywhere between 30 to 60 minutes. Eliminate as many distractions as possible (turn off your phone!).

Pray before you start and when you end. Speak to Jesus as if He were physically present. Remember, He is close and leading you through the process. Be gentle with yourself. Sometimes just knowing you're "surviving the day" shows immense courage and determination.

End your time by thinking on a pleasant memory and thanking God for something. The next day dive back in to continue the process. If unwanted thoughts come outside the scheduled time, tell yourself, "I have other things to do now. I will think about this during my next scheduled time." (Yes, I know that can be a challenge.)

This reminds me of a guy I knew on a S.W.A.T. team. Each day he'd go to the gym with a backpack full of rocks harnessed to himself. He rigorously climbed the "stair-monster." He'd sweat profusely and get red in the face. At the end of an hour, he'd take the backpack off and was done for the day. *Rejoice!* The point is: Over time, he grew stronger and stronger despite the weight of the backpack.

When we can commit to a period of time, we too can start off sweating and getting red in the face, but we will find "joy in the climbing." Always remember: *With loss comes the potential for change and growth.*

The Mourning Process
Transitioning to Post-Traumatic Growth

It is better to go to a house of mourning than to go to a house of feasting.
—Solomon, speaking in Ecclesiastes 7:2

The reality is: We've lost something we can't get back. We have a right to be sad. *It's okay to feel not okay!*

One of things we need to do is separate the *pain* from the *sadness*. Pain is caused by *an event,* which causes *a loss,* which produces *suffering, negative thinking, and emotional torment,* which produces *sadness and grief.* Yet, many of us get stuck in the suffering stage.

It's understandable to feel dejected after a loss. However, if we allow those painful feelings to linger—such as anxiety or anger, they build strength like a snowball that eventually runs out of control—and keeps us from feeling sad, and therefore, healing.

To prevent this, we want to work to *shift our emotional thinking from negative feeling*s such as numbness, anxiety, depression, anger, fear, shame, blame, and rage, to *productive feelings of grief and sadness*. This will enable us to begin to move through the mourning process and helps us adjust better to life—and begin to let go of our toxic coping mechanisms.

Did you know that people cannot feel two opposing emotions at the same time? For example, if someone is relaxed, they can't be anxious; when someone is sad, they can't be mad or bitter.

Things will get better. God has designed us to not stay sad for long periods of time, which is why the emotion of sadness comes and goes like a roller-coaster; it oscillates—sometimes in a flood, other times in a trickle. (A wave of emotion lasts on the average 8 seconds.[91])

God is able to work out a new exciting plan. William Bridges wrote, "All life transitions have a pattern, which if acknowledged will make tough times more comprehensible."

† If you have a hard time knowing how to feel sad, then go back to a time when you remember feeling genuine sadness. For example:

- Remember when your mom or dad forgot your ....
- Remember when you were not chosen for ...

Post-Traumatic Growth

The paradox of trauma is that it has both the power to transform and resurrect.
—Peter A. Levine, PhD

Suffering and sadness are not pathological issues; they are natural and essential parts of living a human life and are also important because they lead to growth.
—Rollo May, PhD

In his book *What Doesn't Kill Us,* Dr. Stephen Joseph found that 43% of people who survived what was considered the worse maritime accident of the 20th century (a passenger ship capsized, instantly plunging passengers and crew into dark, icy waters) said their lives were *better* since the disaster. In psychology this is called "Post-traumatic Growth" (PTG).

PTG refers to positive life changes in the wake of a traumatic or highly challenging event. Both the Bible and science is clear people can and do transform negative predicaments, trauma and loss into personal growth and meaningfulness—a new normal. It's also been called "tragic optimism"—optimism in the face of tragedy. Though we've lost a great deal, we can experience a *"peace that surpasses all understanding"* and a zeal for life."

In 1967, Joni Earikson Tada dove into the Chesapeake Bay after misjudging the shallowness of the water, paralyzing her from the shoulders down. During the first two years of rehabilitation she experienced anger, depression, suicidal thoughts, and doubt in God. Then she learned to paint with a brush between her teeth and began selling her artwork. To date, she has written over 40 books, recorded musical albums, starred in an autobiographical movie of her life, and is an advocate for people with disabilities. Joni experienced PTG.

This is the clincher: PTG doesn't automatically occur as a direct result of trauma. Rather, it's the individual's "constitution" and struggle with the new reality in the aftermath of trauma that determines whether PTG will occur or not. Joni chose to be a survivor, not a victim. And today she loves God more than ever and shares the Gospel news from her wheelchair.

Lucie has recovered from an extremely violent marriage. Not surprising, Lucie struggled with PTSD. She now realizes she was living in a "zombie" state. She didn't think her life was all that bad or different from other people's marital conflicts. One day her mom called and asked her how things were going. Lucie described a vicious marital rape and severe beating she received the day before. She was baffled when two hours later her mom showed up on her doorstep. It was then her loving and supportive mom helped Lucie get support and therapy. She joined a Bible-based abuse recovery group which Lucie describes as her life-line.

Romans 8:37 gives us hope: *"Despite all these things, overwhelming victory is ours through Christ, who loved us."*

Growth occurs when we grapple, confront, engage in a struggle with our pre-conceived beliefs and assumptions; when we search for meaning in the event, and then come to terms with the new reality that follows.

For many people, like myself, who have allowed God's grace and love to enter that hidden, throbbing area of their life, they become *protectors*. It is no accident that there are a great number of survivors in the helping professions (volunteers too). But some, regrettably, become *both protector and predator* as evidenced by stories of abuse at the hands of day care workers, teachers, clergy, nuns, and therapists.

† Here are some PTG questions for you to ask yourself and journal:
- What have I learned so far from enduring suffering?
- To date, what positive changes in myself and my relationships with others, and with God, do I see?

The Examined Life (Restoration Assignments)

Because we survived difficulties that others never faced, we have far more potential than we realize; qualities of resilience, courage, and perseverance. –Brian F. Martin

Talking about loss and the death of a relationship is necessary and healing, but often it's not enough to feel "recovered." I want to give you a few assignments that you can do with God, a recovery partner, or group.

You may be thinking, *I'm doing fine. I've moved beyond my losses and can function quite well.* In your case, there may be no hidden grief. Praise God for that. Some of you have probably learned to manage your losses effectively and are moving forward with life. Yet some you aren't doing so good.

Plato is known for saying, "An unexamined life is not worth living." Before tackling the list of restoration assignments, let me say that we all have different ways of coping with loss and our personal endings. I suggest completing these assignments, but you may choose your own method of coping. Most women find something positive in doing these exercises.

1—*Look at Your Losses*. Recognize there are many intangible losses that occur in chaotic homes and relationships, like losing every child's right to experience a normal loving, protective, and nurturing childhood.

I challenge you to look at your losses to discover what you were robbed of, and then give yourself permission to grieve those losses. (Feeling righteous anger is appropriate.)

Don't forget to include God if your ticked-off or disappointed in Him. Despite our desire to trust Him, sometimes we find there's a feeling of betrayal lingering. Before doing this work, we were controlled by a story we couldn't tell. Not having the words, we went for a coping mechanism, and found ways to express ourselves through those means; or we found ourselves acting in ways we didn't understand.

Part of our healing journey is not only acknowledging our toxic coping mechanisms but letting go of them. Some of us will have to grieve these losses. Write them all down. It's *the first step in acknowledging reality and truth.*

2—*Cry. Tears are medicine.* Crying is a way to get through the pain. Tears, groaning, and waves of grief are normal. When we cry, it appears, stress hormones and toxins are flushed out of our system. We begin to feel calmer, even refreshed.[92]

Washington Irving wrote, "There is a sacredness in tears. They speak more eloquently than ten thousand tongues. They are the messengers of overwhelming grief, and of unspeakable love."

Jesus wept. In His humanity, Jesus felt love, disappointment, loss, agony and sadness—every human emotion that evokes tears from the heart. And Jesus gives His love to us in every imaginable way... even in His tears. The Bible says God collects each tear we cry and will lead us to springs of living water (Isaiah 25:8; Revelation 7:17).

3—*Talk it Out.* I (Kimberly) lost my adolescence and young adulthood, years I could never get back; I could never "talk" to my parents; I lost my virginity to no one special; I submitted to shameful and humiliating behaviors, and never experienced healthy, dating relationships. I always wondered, *Who would I have been? How would my life have been different if I'd followed God's original plan and purpose?* I had every right to cry and mourn for this young girl. I needed safe people to express myself to.

Grievers need to—and most want to—talk about their issues and feelings. We need at least one person we can count on. If a woman has just one person she can count on, she is protected from depression when she experiences significant life stress.[93]

4—*Tell Your Story*. (Review "Finding Your Authentic Voice" on page 17.) Many people begin by writing out their story. Your story can be written either as a narrative account of a few powerful, specific events, or a brief accounting of many events told from your viewpoint, or in the third person, as if it happened to someone else.

With any childhood loss, embrace the wounded little girl. Reacquaint yourself with her. Through your story, give her a sense of safety and connection. You may begin, "What I don't want you to know about me is …" Or begin, "Once upon a time there was a little girl and she …"

Let me add: You may think of this little girl as the one who ruined your family's life or was the "brat." Change this line of thinking to create a loving, caring, and empathetic tone of voice because that is what this little girl always needed. Focus on how the character in the story is thinking and feeling. You were never responsible for the hurt, but you are responsible for seeking the Healer.

5—*Write an Acceptance Letter*. This is the conclusion to the story you wrote; your testimony. Every story or article has a conclusion which summarizes and ties the written material all together. *Acceptance* is a crucial element in *finalizing* your ending. Can you say, "My life didn't go as planned and that's okay."? I believe you've come to grips with your tragic circumstances and have accepted reality. Finish your story by completing these sentences.

- This is what happened ...
- This is what I did to survive it ...
- This has been the cost ...
- This is what I've learned ...
- This is how I choose to respond to life now ...
- My purpose in life for now is to ...
- When I look back on my life, the evidence I see of God's love, grace, and mercy bringing me to where I am today is evident ...

Try this exercise: To inspire others, imagine you are the focus of a documentary, "Women Who Survived PTS and Abuse." You are asked, "Tell me what strengths and how your faith in God have helped you survive." Write out your answer.

As you have been diligently working through all these exercises you have been converting toxic negative feelings to feelings of sadness, which has been a major goal. Now is time to convert the sadness to purpose.

6—*Convert the pain and sadness to purpose.* Before I talked about converting toxic negative feelings to feelings of sadness. There's nothing wrong with feeling sad, but we don't want to stay sad. We want to convert it to purpose.

As a child, actress Halle Berry watched her mother being brutally beaten by her father. Yet she was able to achieve success in a competitive field. Bill Clinton was traumatized by violence in his home. He found a way to turn that fear into confidence—enough to lead the nation for 8-years. Oprah Winfrey, Christina Aguilera, Drew Barrymore, and countless other women and men have turned their stories of abuse into success stories. At some point you will want to use your story and talk about it. You can never say you've wasted your life. Your story can be empowering and healing.

When the Holy Spirit tells you that you're ready, use your story to help others. Viktor Frankl wrote, "In some ways suffering ceases to be suffering at the moment it finds a meaning."

It's been said that those who suffer the most, change the world the most. God supplies comfort, hope, love, encouragement, mercy, knowledge, and faith first to you for your own healing and spiritual growth. He then provides these things *through you* for helping others.

Susannah wrote, "At the time I didn't know. Now I do. I wouldn't take back that terrible experience for anything. Too much light has come out of my darkness." Anyone who has experienced pain and sadness has the capacity to respond with empathy and compassion towards another wounded and downcast person.

Pain and sorrow can have a purpose. Milton Erikson said, "It is really amazing what people can do. Only they don't know what they can do." Ask God to show you what makes you come alive—then go and pursue it.

Don't let anything stop you! Let your pain motivate you to serve another, helping someone else make it through. Invest in something that can give satisfaction and fulfillment. For example, become an advocate against domestic violence or a mentor. God will do with you, and in you, what He's not doing with any other person. That's exciting!

7—*Convert sad feelings to grateful feelings.* Practice gratitude and make it a conscious everyday effort. Count your wins for the day and thank God. It's no secret that people who are grateful are healthier, happier, and more optimistic. Every day answer, *"What are three things I'm most grateful for today?"* This results in peace, and we open up new neural pathways in our brains for productive thinking and change. We feel so much better!

Dealing with Anniversary Dates and/or Triggers: Even after all the work you've done, certain occasions, dates, places, smells, for example, will still make you sad, and can certainly re-trigger the pain you felt. There is a temptation to try to handle these times or dates alone, or stuff your feelings back down—don't. This is normal. Turn to Jesus first. Then find your recovery partner or someone to help you process through your feelings.

† † †

I'm asking you to do a lot. These exercises are tough. I want you to have plenty of ammunition for fighting the pain, sorrow and lies that have been the landscape of your life. I also want you to feel hopeful that by experiencing both the painful emotions of grief and mourning *and* the positive feelings of purpose and rebuilding, that you can heal from your wounds of abuse.

You may fear you may go crazy—you won't. With God at your side you'll be able to get through the work. He may also lead you to a Christian counselor if it becomes too overwhelming. You could experience some physical symptoms like stomachaches, insomnia, headaches—don't ignore them; they're a sign of emotionally healing. Symptoms will subside over time. It's always a good idea to have a doctor check you out. Work at your own pace. Don't give up, which is what the enemy desires you to do. *You are already an overcomer!* Let's now see how *ready, willing* and *able* you are to implement these suggestions.

† How *important* would you say it is for you to follow through with some of these exercises?

Joy Comes in the 'Mourning'

Psalm 30:5 says, *"Weeping may endure for a night, but joy comes in the morning."* Ever wonder what constitutes a "night"? Second Peter 3:8 tells us, *"With the Lord a day is like a thousand years."* In other words, a night be a literal night, or it may be years.

So far in this study, we've been made aware of the transformative power of pain, but we don't know much about joy. Joy comes after we've done the dark side and we're ready to move into the light. But often, we feel we need permission to feel joy and fulfilment.

My wise friend Annie Paden, author of *Fruit Flies,* writes,

> Joy can run deep, sort of like a submarine, beneath the waves of our circumstances, but given enough time it will surface. You may not be able to feel it for a season, but given enough time, it will surface. It may be a long season, but God has not forgotten you, and His joy is alive.

God doesn't intend us to continuously mourn. He wants us to enjoy the beauty of life He's created. God repeatedly calls us to grow through suffering trials. *"Be happy and full of joy, because the Lord has done a wonderful thing"* (Joel 2:21, NEV).

Now it's time to give yourself permission to feel joy. God created us to think great and positive things, yet, we seem to resist them. Don't let your head battle against it.

There's nothing wrong with desiring happiness. Psalm 37:4 says, *"Delight yourself in the LORD, and he will give you the desires of your heart."* That's our objective: to delight ourselves in God. Nothing short of this will bring us true joy.

Joy is what we're entitled to. I challenge you to remember the last time you felt joyful. Then, with God's help, create a vision of what a joyful future looks like to you. Hang onto it to that picture!

8

HUSTLING FOR OUR WORTHINESS

Later that day the voting took place, and Mr. Zeigler told me how proud he was that my title had won. I soaked it up like a sponge. I hadn't been told anything positive for so long that I nearly cried. At the end of the day, after assuring me that I wasn't in trouble, Mr. Zeigler gave me a letter to take to Mother.

Elated, I ran to Mother's house faster than ever before. As I should have expected, my happiness was short lived. The b---- tore the letter open, read it quickly and scoffed, "Well, Mr. Zeigler says I should be proud of you for naming the school newspaper. He also claims that you are one of the top pupils in his class. Well, aren't you special!" Suddenly, her voice turned ice cold and the jabbed finger at my face hissed, "Get one thing straight, you little b-----! There is nothing you can do to impress me! Do you understand me? You are a *nobody!* An *it!* You are a bastard child! I hate you and wish you were dead! *Dead!*

After tearing the letter into tiny pieces, Mother returned to her television show. I stood motionless, gazing at the letter which lay like snowflakes at my feet. This time the word "*It*" stunned me like never before. She had stripped me of my very existence. I gave all I could to accomplish anything positive for *her* recognition. But again, I failed. I knelt down, trying to put the pieces of the letter back together. It was impossible. I dumped them in the trash, wishing my life would end. I truly believed, at any moment, that death would be better. I was nothing but an *It*.[94] –Dave Pelzer, *A Child Called It*

Hopefully, you were never called an "It." Yet, most likely there are certain names or labels you've been wearing as your identity. When you look into your mirror each day, what statements about yourself are reflected back to you?

If you're like most survivors, the "you" that you experience is not the real "you." If you were abused as a child or teen, your logical thinking center was not developed until adulthood. You couldn't logically sort out truth from deception. You wrongly believed what your abuser told you, which became true as far as you were concerned and never challenged.

If you are an adult in an abusive relationship, your thought process has been invaded by a manipulator. One minute you may be told your stupid, fat, and ugly; later, you're sexy and smart. Abusers undermine a person's self-worth and identity.

What we believe about ourselves is not necessarily the truth.

The toxic labels we give ourselves are swirling around in our minds, what I call our *inner abuser:* the unconscious voice that calls us names today: *incompetent, ugly, fat, stupid, unlovable, worthless.* *"If I were only smarter, stronger, or likeable, then ...."*

In chapter one, when I wrote of the verbal abuser, I pointed out that Proverbs 15:4 speaks about the destructive power of words as having *"the power of life and death"* and *"crushes the spirit."* We too have the ability to speak life or death to ourselves. Too many of us are presently speaking death, which must change.

The inner turmoil will continue to lower our self-worth and intrude unless we get rid of the inner abuser. It's not easy and it takes time. But God's power can prevail.

† Memorize this: *I am the one who decides if another person's statement about me has power over me or not. Me only.*

Think of the verbal abuse you've experienced. In what way was the treatment you received milder compared to how you verbally abuse yourself? (The same applies to physical abuse too.)

You Have Forgotten Who You Are

A procession of angels pass before a human being where he or she goes, proclaiming, "Make way for the image of God." –Joshua be Levi

In the classic Disney movie, *The Lion King,* Simba's dead father says to Simba, "You have forgotten who you are and so have forgotten me. Look inside yourself, Simba. You are more than what you have become. You must take your place in the Circle of Life."

God says, "You are more than you think you are." God always sees us as we can be, not as we are. Our real self hasn't died. It's just gone underground. There's nothing we can do to establish our worth. It's already been established by our Creator. Scripture tells us:

God created man in his own image, in the image of God he created him; male and female he created them. God blessed them ...God saw all that he had made, and it was very good (Genesis 1:27-28; 31).

A Randy Glasbergen comic goes, "Your resume here says that you are created in the image of God. Very impressive!"

When God made every human being, Scripture says, *"God saw all that he had made, and it was very good" (Genesis 1:31).* In other words, *you* have been made "very good" and "excellent in every way." You wear a spiritual label, "Handmade by the Lord." God wants us to not only know the wonder of being made in His image, but to experience it at a soul level.

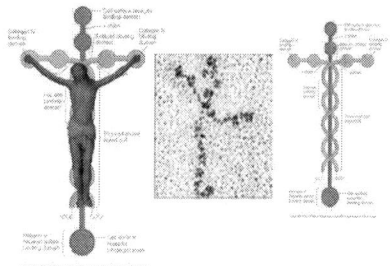

God is the choreographer and author of our genetic code, DNA, language, and every cell in each organ. One remarkable example is "laminin." Laminin is a cell with significant characteristics that stump and awe most of us. It's a *glycoprotein* that holds the human being together ... and it looks like a crucifix. Laminin's physical properties are also symbolic. Isn't that awesome! (BTW: *Yeshua* is translated "Jesus.")

Resurrecting Your True Self
God's Word says if we belong to Christ, we are a brand-new person. *The old life is gone; a new life has begun!" (2 Corinthians 5:17)* We get a life do-

over. This means Jesus has the power to change our identity. We learn we're not who we thought we were supposed to be, or who we pictured ourselves being. We come to the place where we recognize that our value is not dependent on other people's opinions, or performance, titles, appearance, achievement, or who we know.

The phrase "Christ in me" is used quite often in the Bible (John 14:20; 17:23; Galatians 2:20). Our worth comes from our *position* in Christ—not our *condition* in this world. The recurrent phrase "in Christ" means Christ's power is *in us*, which means we have Him and His power which is working to transform us. It also means there is Love and Beauty within us. Every day we need to be reminded of who we really are; that "Christ in me" is waiting to be expressed.

The greatest sadness is the ignorance or disbelief of one's true self. It breaks my heart when women look at God's creation and think, 'Wow! God is astonishing!' but then look in the mirror and say *ugly!* as if He didn't create both. We're not defined by the things we suffered or the labels which have been put on us. We are not our weakness, our addictions, nor our anger, shame, fear, or depression.

† Say: *I am unique and a radiant center of personality and feelings. I have the courage to be myself and not like everybody else. I am a living, vibrant, magnificent image of Jesus Christ.*

"Jesus Plus Nothing"

Guide me in your truth and teach me. – Psalm 25:5

Many of us never realized until now just how much someone else, even our culture, has regulated our life and daily choices. *Every single one of us struggles with the oppression of being devalued.* We were created to receive our identity from God, but today are caught up with creating multiple identities from other people and sources.

One source is social media. For example, on Facebook we can mask who we are and project how we wish to be seen. We can boast a thousand friends and never truly be known. We can follow others and think we're relevant, all the while we're falling away from our true selves believing *I am only as good as the number of "Likes" I get on Facebook and Instagram.*

"Acceptance" means we seek the approval and/or favor from another human being. For most of us, including myself, we desire to feel accepted by others. Validation fills the void. After all, God created us to belong to a community. Too many of us measure ourselves on the "favorable reception" ruler.

In his book, *Dealing with the Rejection and Praise of Men,* Bob Sorge is direct and doesn't back down from his point of view,

> When we realize we are accepted and embraced by the great God of the universe, the acceptance of people becomes secondary. All I really need is His acceptance. When I have that, I can face rejection from anyone. This is how Jesus lived. He had the Father's acceptance so He didn't need anyone else's to give Him a sense of self-identity. When the Father said, *"This is my Son, whom I love; with him I am well pleased"* (Matthew 3:17), I can imagine Jesus's heart response being something like, *"That's all I need! Just to know You approve of My life, Father, is enough for Me. Now I am complete and can rest in Your affection and approval. I don't care who rejects Me, as long as I know You accept Me!"* Jesus knew He couldn't depend upon the acceptance of man, for men are fickle in their fallenness. The only acceptance that Jesus allowed to feed His spirit was the Father's.
>
> As long as we look to flesh and blood for our approval, we will be snared by seasons of frustration and disappointment. My message is: *Jesus plus nothing.* When I have Him, I truly need nothing else. When I have His endorsement, I need no one else's. When I have His approval, I need no other source. His acceptance alone is enough.
>
> I am not advocating an independent spirit. The Lord has called us to walk in inter-dependence with fellow Christians. We need other members. We look to each other for encouragement, counsel, prayer support, practical help, wisdom, perspective, for correction, etc. But we ought not look for others to be our sole source of acceptance. That comes from God alone. It is a sign of maturity when we can receive

correction without interpreting it as rejection and not allowing myself to be penetrated by your rejection.[95]

† How should this information impact the way you think about yourself? What does it reveal to about God's character?

Complete in Him

In Him you have been made complete ... –Paul, speaking in Colossians 2:10

Let's say your earthly dad has rejected you most of your life. ("Rejection" can mean *abandonment, refusing to recognize, cast out, discarding as useless, denied* or *renounced.*) You still wear the battle wounds because no matter how hard you tried to get his favor, all you got was rejection upon rejection. As a "good Christian" you chose to forgive your dad. Then you see him at a family gathering. As is his nature, he is emotionally abusive, tearing you down. Now every wound from the past gets ripped up all over again. Once again, you're back in that place of feeling crushed, depressed and rejected by dad.

Maybe this scenario happens when your ex-husband picks up your kids for the weekend. There are hordes of scenarios where this happens. The critical question is: *To whom are you looking as the source of your acceptance?* It may be a number of people depending on your role. For example, when you are in the role of wife and mother, you may be looking for your husband's approval. When you are a student, you may be looking for your teacher's acceptance. Or, when you're at church, it may be your pastor's approval.

I encourage you today to unreservedly receive God's acceptance. When our heavenly Father approves of us, then other people can call us names and tell us how bad we are and it won't wound because our spirit is being nurtured and fed by the Father's Spirit.

This is a great challenge for each one of us, including me. We can get there if we remain connected to God. The key is deciding that He is going to be our sole source of acceptance.

Scripture tells us that we are "complete" in Him (Colossians 2:9-10). When the Bible tells us we're "complete," it's saying that when Christ comes into our lives, He fills us completely with Him; we lack nothing. We don't need anyone or anything else to complete us.

How can this happen? When we choose Jesus as our Lord and Savior, He hits the *restart* button. Everything we've done—past, present, and even future—has been forgiven and nailed to the cross, making us "complete." We are immediately a new creation (2 Corinthians 5:17). The truth: *"You were dead because of your sins and because your sinful nature was not yet cut away. Then God made you alive with Christ, for he forgave all our sins. He canceled the record of the charges against us and took it away by nailing it to the cross" (Colossians 2:13-14).*

Recognize: If man's acceptance will build you up, then man's rejection will tear you down. It appears then *the only way to close the door to another person's rejection is by closing the door to needing and depending upon another person's acceptance and praise.*

Jesus said, *"No one can serve two masters. Either he will hate the one and love the other, or he will be devoted to the one and despise the other" (Matthew 6:24).* No one can get through life on other people's praises. We must choose whose voice is more important: God or man.

† Consider today who is your master? Name the people you are looking to as the source of your acceptance.

The Snare of Praise

It is better to take refuge in the LORD than to trust in man. –Psalm 118:8

I (Kimberly) couldn't believe what I had just heard. In 2009 a producer from the *Focus on the Family Weekend* radio program informed me I'd be one of their featured speakers in the near future. Naturally, I was ecstatic. Then I learned the feature was to be delayed, possibly cancelled, not once, but twice. Was the devil working in the background or was God the one putting up the obstacles because it wasn't the right time? Perhaps I simply wasn't ready for this kind of exposure.

I finally taped the interview with the host Bill Maher and it ran one Saturday morning on the radio. The segment was released on CD. As I held that little piece of plastic, I beamed with pride. *Praise God! Thank you, Lord!* There's something intoxicating about seeing your name in print and having it known by others. I tasted it for just a moment.

When the taped interview wrapped up, Mr. Maher did not mention my book or myself as a resource. *What's wrong with me? Why is my book not good enough to mention like with your other guests?* In that moment, I felt the sting of the worse kind of rejection—because the praise I'd been seeking vaporized.

Do you realize that rejection and praise are at the opposite ends of the same continuum but with *identical roots*? Pastor Sorge said, "Those who fear the rejection of man have a deep yearning for the praise of man and set their souls up for repetitive heartache."[96]

We might call this person a "people-pleaser" or "perfectionist." She thinks: *I must be loved or approved by every significant person in my life. I depend on others for my value; I must be painstakingly competent and perfect in order to receive praise and thereby consider myself worthwhile.*

It's been said for every one positive comment made; a child receives 10 negative comments; it takes 7 compliments to undo the effects of just one criticism. No wonder we grow up feeling we need to do whatever it takes to be accepted. We thrive on praise. This is expressed in Proverbs 29:25, *"The fear of human opinion disables; trusting in God protects you from that" (MSG).*

If we are living to make sure others like us, we give them the power to determine our self-worth. I must constantly remind myself I work for God, not people. I can't allow other people's approval or disapproval of me dominate my thinking. That's a stronghold.

Our nature desires to be noticed and seen. The issue is, once again, that God desires we first receive praise from Him (John 5:44; Acts 5:29; Gal. 1:10). The Bible cautions us against seeking man's admiration. First, people are fickle. One minute they love you, the next they turn their back to you. Even Christians eventually disappoint. Secondly, when we stand before God at the end of our lives, other people's opinions won't matter a bit. Only God's opinion will be relevant (2 Corinthians 10:18).

How then do we receive encouragement and accolades from the Father? Let me suggest:

1—*Let Him speak to you through His Word* as you study the Bible. When we pray, we speak to God, but when we study the Scriptures, God speaks to us. Second Timothy 3:16 tells us, *"the whole Bible was given to us by inspiration from God and is useful to teach us what is true ..."*

2—*Pray and listen* for His quiet voice to speak into your mind.

3—*Discern proper praise from other people.* God has made us to need encouragement from each other. He will speak through others who build you up, versus tear you down (Hebrews 3:13; Romans 14:19; 1 Thess. 3:2). When Jesus affirmed His disciples, He didn't gush all over them to keep them propped up emotionally. When He praised them, it was very strategic: He affirmed what God was doing through them.

Pastor Sorge wrote, "I do not seek the praise of other people, but I do seek to honor and encourage other believers as much as possible."[97] Never forget this truth: *"The LORD is for me, so I will have no fear. What can mere people do to me?" (Psalm 118:6)*

† Finish each of these sentences:
- When people compliment me, I feel ...
- I feed off other people's praise because ...
- Seeking God's praise instead of another's feels to me like ...

Shame Off You!

Guard my life and rescue me; do not let me be put to shame, for I take refuge in you.
—Psalm 25:20

One night I (Kimberly) met up with a guy friend at a bar. As usual I'd begun my journey to getting plastered. He took me to a small party at some dude's apartment where we continued to booze it up. I was led into a bedroom by one of the guys. Wasted and barely conscious, I didn't realize until hours later that four guys raped me.

The word spread like wild fire in the college dorm that I "pulled a train" (when a group of males, one after the other, have sex with a woman). My guy friend didn't stand up for me, and my peers ostracized and ignored me, presuming I "wanted it." To them, and to me, the only difference between me and a prostitute is I didn't exchange money. I felt covered inside and out with the vomit of humiliation and shame, and it wouldn't wash off no matter how many showers I took.

I don't know which felt worse—feeling defiled from the "gang rape" or the social judgment. Both were bad. Emotionally frozen, my only recourse was to keep this horrid incident a secret. Eventually I just became numb to being used and thrown out. The way I felt was the way I acted. (I'm so glad this happened before phone cameras!)

What I've done is horrible. I'm a bad person; hideous and worthless. It's no secret. I'm naked for everyone to stare at. I'm ignored as if I don't exist. I have no value to those whose opinions matter most. Like a play, the curtain parted and my neurosis appeared center stage for all to see.

Shame is the most toxic human emotion and our biggest threat to accepting our identity as God's child.

It's been said that if you tell a lie long enough it becomes a truth. *Shame comes out of a lie someone told you about yourself—a lie that you were 'less than.'* And this lie has become your truth. An FBI agent, specializing in behavioral analysis, wrote, "Most people—both laypersons and professionals—are not very good at detecting lies. Identifying deceit is so difficult. ... Truth is essential for all relations."[98]

Think about this: If we didn't long to be wanted and loved, then we wouldn't care. If we didn't care, then we couldn't be shamed by other's rejection or attacks.

And the shame of sexual abuse is the worst because your internal organs, and your very soul, are invaded. Being used for someone else's sexual gratification is humiliating and demeaning; it kills the soul. A naked body is so intimate that when violated it brings on overwhelming levels of shame. Let us not forget that Jesus identifies with all victims who feel the shame of nakedness. (If you are a victim of sexual abuse, please read and work through the chapter titled "Sexual Shame Off You!")

Shame is not the same as guilt or humiliation or embarrassment. Humiliation and embarrassment don't afflict a person's soul. People believe they deserve their shame; they don't believe they deserve humiliation. And with embarrassment, you eventually laugh about it. With shame, you never laugh.

Typically, *guilt* is a result of something *we do*. It's a valuable signal indicating a wrong or bad behavior. Whereas *shame* is a result of something *done to us* by another person. There's a big difference between *I failed* (guilt), and *I'm a failure* (shame.)

The difference lies in the way we talk to ourselves. Shame focuses on self; guilt on behavior. Guilt always relates to the past (I did bad), whereas shame brings the feeling into the present (I am bad).

† Your shame all started with one lie you were told about yourself. It's a fact: *God doesn't make junk!* Those who spoke words of death over you and broke your heart were liars! Can you name that lie?

Clarify Ownership

Healing occurs when we bring the toxic emotion of shame out of the dark closet, giving words to it, and then begin the process of eliminating it. Once we recognize the shame and lies, we've been carrying, the next step is to figure out who is responsible.

In my story, *who is at fault? Who needs to take ownership for hurting another human being; for assaulting an image-bearer of God?* The rapists were responsible. So why do we turn it the other way around? One reason: When a person submits to the control of another person for a sufficient period of time, it slowly erodes her self-identity, and the ability to think and reason for herself. She begins to think through the eyes of the controlling person, rather than with her own mind.

It's like the boiling frog story: place a frog in boiling water, it will jump out. But if you place it in cold water that is slowly heated, it won't perceive the danger and will be cooked to death.

Consider what Jesus, the greatest therapist who ever lived, said:

The things that come out of the mouth come from the heart, and these make a man 'unclean.' For out of the heart come evil thoughts, murder, adultery, sexual immorality, theft, false testimony, slander. These are what make a man 'unclean' (Matthew 15:18-20).

The good man brings good things out of the good stored up in his heart, and the evil man brings evil things out of the evil stored up in his heart. For out of the overflow of his heart his mouth speaks (Luke 6:45).

Some people torment us into believing we're dirty, unworthy, to blame, and unacceptable to God and to others. In biblical times, this condition was called "unclean." Today we call a person who is using "unclean." This is not the context in which it's meant.

Unclean translated means "impure." Impurities—emotional or chemical—pollute the body and desecrate God's temple, which is us. In the Old Testament, one of the things God considered "unclean" was death, and throughout the book of Leviticus we read that contact with death brings uncleanliness. How appropriate since abuse brings about death.

In this Scripture Jesus is saying: *It's not what goes in my mouth that defiles me; it's what comes out of my mouth and heart that defiles me.* The mouth reveals most clearly the condition of the heart, and thereby behavior.

Therefore, if another person spews their verbal vomit onto me—calls me a *blah ... blah ... blah*, they cannot destroy my soul with their tongue, or make me feel contaminated because the verbal vomit came out of *their* mouth; it came out of *their* heart.

Jesus said, *"Don't be afraid of those who want to kill your body; they cannot touch your soul"* (Matthew 10:28). The only thing that can dirty me is what comes from inside of my heart. According to Jesus:

An abuser = Unclean. A victim/survivor = Clean.

When we love another person, and that person has power and authority over us, we tend to take the person's "unclean" dirty words and internalize them; believe they are truth.

Remember: The heart is connected to the mouth. Only if the heart is changed, can the words which come out of the mouth change. And recall what I asked you earlier to memorize: *I am the one who decides if another person's statement about me has power over me or not. Me only.*

† Explain in your own words what Jesus's therapeutic words of wisdom taught you. Describe what "clean" means to you.

Investigate the Truth: Already Clean

No one and nothing can make you an outcast, dirty, or untouchable. People can't; the sins of your family can't; abusers can't. –Edward T. Welch, PhD

Decades ago when my (Kimberly) dad called me a "fat piggy" I internalized and believed it. My thinking errors were:

- I'm ashamed.
- I'm unlovable.
- I'm ugly; my body is awful.

Healing meant changing my shame-talk and investigating this statement. *Was it true?* I believed it was. *Could I be absolutely certain it was true?* Upon further investigation, I recognized I was a little overweight, but I'd never been a "fat piggy." I was "clean." Dad's critical labels made him unclean—not anything I did or ate.

Other people's evil words only taint themselves and make them dirty.
Jesus said,

> *You are already clean because of the word I have spoken to you. Remain in me, as I also remain in you. No branch can bear fruit by itself; it must remain in the vine. Neither can you bear fruit unless you remain in me (John 15:3-4).*

(In biblical times agriculture was the mainstay which is why Jesus and others use so many gardening and farming illustrations.)

What a beautiful description of *your* personal relationship with Christ! You connecting with Jesus; He connecting with you. Let's break this down. To "remain" or "abide" in Jesus is to be rooted and grounded and filled with Him. The result: We are part of Him. We are one. We are clean.

What is your response? Do you really believe what Jesus says is truth? If yes, then *you* are "clean." Remain connected to Jesus and you'll continue to be clean and pure—free from any kind of contamination.

In this parable, we are the branch—the branch attached to Jesus, the vine. According to *Vines Complete Expository Dictionary,* the word "fruit" means "the visible expression of Christ's power working inwardly and invisibly" inside of me. So, let's read it again in this context: *To receive the visible expression of Christ's power working inwardly and invisibly in you; you must remain in Jesus Christ.*

In other words, when I connect with Christ, His power will be at work in me. I will produce good stuff, not bad stuff. In biblical terms, I'm a "good tree." Jesus said, *"A good tree cannot bear bad fruit, and a bad tree cannot bear good fruit" (Matthew 7:18).*

- Fact: You are connected to Jesus.
- Fact: You are clean.
- Fact: You are the image of "good fruit" and a "good tree;" of goodness, not sin!

Let this sink in: Even if you've had contact with an unclean person, as a believer in Jesus Christ and His Word, *you cannot bear bad or evil things!* Second Corinthians 5:17 confirms that *you are a new creation in Christ.* You are no longer the same person. You have been made new spiritually by the power of God. In time, your emotions and relationships will follow.

Grasping the truth of Jesus's words doesn't change what happened, but it does change our *perceptions* of the event; it doesn't rewrite the past, but it does rewrite the brain by rewriting a shame-based sense of self.

Let me conclude this teaching with another Jesus truth. He said, *"... on the day of judgment people will give an account for every careless word they speak ... (Matthew 12:36).*

† Try holding your thoughts for at least 12 minutes on one or two of these Scriptures, in these two sections, each day for the next month. Ponder what God's Word is teaching you about yourself, about Him, and any feelings of shame. Jesus has a lot to say.

Shame Which Comes from Our Actions

One's dignity may be assaulted, vandalized and cruelly mocked, but it cannot be taken away unless it's surrendered. –actor Michael J. Fox in *Saving Milly*

Unprocessed trauma can cause people to react to their world through emotions, beliefs and physical sensations that were present at the time of their earlier traumatic experiences. Some act out the pain, rage, hate or despair and don't care who gets hurt. They become sharp-tongued, rude, or abusive. They get caught in the same web of sin that caught the person who abused them. Others don't understand that what they're doing is wrong and wounding. They may choose illegal or addictive behaviors in order to cope, such as shoplifting, drug abuse or compulsive behaviors.

Shame is not only a product of what others have done to you, it's also a product of what you've done to yourself and others; a result of breaking God's laws. A *New Yorker* cartoon shows a woman seated in a witness box saying, "I know he beat me because of his childhood abuse, but I shot him because of mine."

Psychological explanations can be immensely helpful in recovery work, but they're not helpful when they invite people to avoid being fully accountable for the harmful consequences of their decisions. You may have found that the more unmanageable the guilt and shame become, the more difficult it is to admit to the wrongdoing, even feel remorse.

What we learn about Jesus in the Bible is He reinforced the idea that people should take responsibility for their own actions and lives. We need to go to God with our own baggage. We confess our wrongdoings and ask for His forgiveness, which He grants immediately.

We choose to take responsibility and *repent,* which means we feel sorrow for our offensive actions and resolve not to act in the same way again; to go in a new direction. Another word is *atone,* which means to repair an injury and work toward restoring the wrong that's been done. If possible, we *take accountability and make amends* with anyone we've afflicted, offended, or avoided.

I also suggest *redirecting your viewpoint.* For example, if you're feeling guilty about a situation, maybe it wasn't entirely your fault? Did you do the best you could under the circumstances? Would someone else in your position have responded the exact same way?

† Pray Psalm 51:1-2: *"Have mercy on me, O God, according to your unfailing love; according to your great compassion blot out my transgressions. Wash away all my iniquity and cleanse me from my sin."*

G.R.O.W. [God Restores Our Worth]

When people pursue an identity apart from God, it leads to confusion.
—Caroline Leaf, PhD

A fable goes: A mother tiger died giving birth to a cub. A pack of goats came upon the baby tiger and invited the cub to join the pack. As months went by the baby cub took on all the characteristics of a goat, even though he was a tiger by nature.

One day the king tiger came through the forest where the pack of goats lived. He stumbled across the tiger that was acting like a silly goat. He roared, "What is the meaning of this masquerade? Why are you behaving in such a different way?"

All the cub knew was to bleat and nibble at the grass. Then the king tiger figured out the problem: *This little creature has no idea who he is!* The king took him to the river and let him see for the first time a reflection of himself. "See. You are not really a goat. You are one of us." Then he said, "Follow me, little one. I will help you become the grand thing you were created to be!"

Want a shot of immunity against criticism and rejection? Let your Creator show you your true nature; let Him show you that you are a worthy person deserving of love and approval regardless of what someone else has told you. Finding out how you've been designed and how God feels about you may be the most surprising discovery you'll ever make. Get ready for a paradigm shift!

The Power of "I Am" Exercise

Have you ever *really* thought about the power of the words "I am"? Do you truly recognize the subconscious "I am" statements that you are holding about yourself?

"I am" is one of the most powerful statements we can make. It's more powerful than "I have" or "I can." Whatever follows "I am" starts the creation of it.

Numerous times both God and Jesus used "I am" statements about themselves. God told Moses His name is "I Am" (Exodus 3:14). They were making a powerful claim pointing to their divinity.

Obviously, we're not professing to be God, but when we make a claim "I am ..." we are claiming *to be* a person of worthiness. When

God is within us we become the best possible version of ourselves, and we have the honor of revealing God to the world.

For the next month, take one statement a day from the list of scriptural statements and meditate on it; grapple with it; study it; visualize it as reality. *Then write out all the evidence to support this belief.* Journal your feelings, even body sensations; write out a prayer. Apply what you've learned from the five steps.

For example, the first one is: "I am beautiful."

- This is true because God says so.
- My neighbor told me I was so kind to bring her flowers from my garden. She said, "You're beautiful."
- My heart is no longer hardened towards certain people. This makes me beautiful (inside beauty).

Then complete this sentence: "Because [*the statement*] this means I can … For example: Because *I am beautiful*, I can walk into the room exuding confidence.

Positive Beliefs About Yourself

- I am beautiful (Song of Songs).
- I am radiant (Psalm 34:4).
- I have the highest possible value (Psalm 8:5; Genesis 1:27).
- I am fearfully ("awesome") and brilliantly made (Psalm 139:14).
- I am born of God. The evil one cannot touch me (1 John 5:18).
- I am the apple of God's eye (Deuteronomy 32:10).
- I am a beloved child (Ephesians 5:1).
- I have a mind like Jesus Christ (1 Corinthians 2:16).
- I am God's child and Christ's friend (John 1:12; 15:15).
- I am forgiven; my sins have been taken away (Romans 3:23-24).
- I am free from condemnation (Romans 8:1-2).
- I am a conqueror (*a survivor*; Romans 8:37).
- I am a saint (1 Corinthians 1:2).
- My heart has been cleansed from a guilty conscious (Heb. 10:22).

- I am holy, blameless, covered with God's love (Ephesians 1:4).
- I am transformed (*sanctified*) by God's presence (Ephesians 1:1).
- I have the favor of God (Proverbs 8:35)
- I am the salt and light of the earth (Matthew 5:13-14).
- I am God's adopted child (Ephesians 1:5-6).
- I am God's work of art; His masterpiece (Ephesians 2:10).
- I have direct access to God (Ephesians 2:18; 3:12).
- I am confident because of God's work in me (Philippians 1:6).
- I can do anything through Christ's strength (Philippians 4:13).

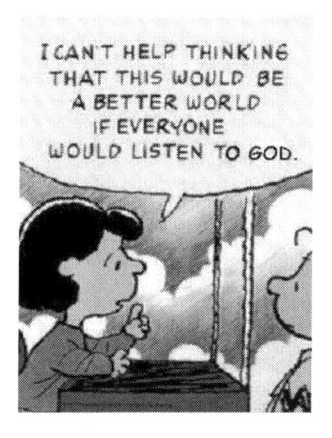

Don't worry if you can't fully grasp these truths about yourself; no one can at first. We may intellectually get it, and believe God said it, but do we experience these truths about ourselves and act on them? In many cases, no. Through practice and Scripture meditation, God's Word can re-route our thinking patterns. We can pair our negative thinking belief with the truth of Scripture, thereby, *creating a new memory*.

Healing Exercises

1—*Write a goodbye letter to the woman you are leaving behind.* Then write another letter to your current self from your future self (choose the time frame: 6 months; 1 year; or 5 years in the future). *Where are you? What are you doing? Describe how well you are doing.*

2— *Address the child or the young girl or woman you were when you were being abused.* Tell her she didn't do anything wrong; she wasn't bad, but what was done to her was bad. Tell her something like:

- You did the best you could.
- You faced a situation (situations) no child/young girl/woman should ever have to endure.

- You didn't understand what was happening or being done to you.
- You were in pain and suffered, but you survived.
- You don't deserve to carry shame and guilt. Those emotions belong to the abuser, not you.
- You are lovable.

Hear God saying to her, "I love you. You're not alone. You have me. Together we'll heal the wounds and get through this. I will give you the power and inner strength to do it."

3—*Balloon Exercise:* One of the interactive exercises I do a is give each woman a balloon and marker.

- Blow up the balloon and draw your face on it.
- Stand up and silently recall the biggest shame-based lie you have believed and share it with God.
- I say: "On the count of three, sit down and bust the balloon—*bust the lie.* 1-2-3! Satan's domain over this lie has now been broken!" Then rejoice and celebrate!

Warning: If you do this in a church or retreat center, warn the person in charge. The first time I did this exercise, a manager rushed into the room thinking he heard gun shots! If doing this is not possible, take out a piece of paper, write your lies on it, then tell Satan his domain over this lie will now be broken—then destroy the paper!

Pretty Woman

Vivian: *People put you down enough, you start to believe it.*
Edward Lewis: *I think you are a very bright, very special woman.*
Vivian: *The bad stuff is easier to believe. You ever notice that?*
—dialogue from the movie *Pretty Woman*

You've probably seen the ultimate chick flick movie *Pretty Woman*. Vivian (played by Julia Roberts), a small-time prostitute, hits it big when she falls in love with her client, Edward Lewis (played by

Richard Gere). Edward is transformed by real love. He made Vivian an offer that logic would dictate she should accept. He'll be her "Sugar Daddy," and put her in a high-class condo with a running credit card tab, just as long as she's there for him when he comes to town. She'll be his "Sugar Baby" mistress.

In the week they've been together, Vivian has changed. She's shed her shame and image as a prostitute. She sees herself as the pretty woman she is, with more to offer a man than her body.

She tells Edward that when she was a little girl, her mother locked her up in the attic when she was bad. She'd pretend she was a princess in a tower, and a knight would come to rescue her.

Vivian's vintage line: "Never in all that time did the knight say, 'Honey, I'll put you up in a great condo.' A few months ago, I could have taken your offer. Now something is different. I want more!"

I love this story. It's the quintessential story of the beautiful warrior woman proclaiming, "I will not accept your crumbs." Her image of the worthless victim, amidst a hard and unfair world, waiting for her prince to rescue and take care of her is replaced with "I am a somebody." Jesus constantly associated with people who were considered nobody's—the "bad" or "unclean" like prostitutes and tax collectors—sinners. He never thought of them as bad or worthless. He condemned the sinful behavior, but never the sinner.

To Jesus, every person had the ability to turn their lives around and have a relationship with God. He constantly invited people into a relationship with Him because He knew *connecting with Him* is what gave them the power to be who He created them to do.

Open your eyes to see the sin in the person who wounded or abused you—not the other way around. If you were a Vivian, recognize you can be forgiven for prostitution; recognize you too were a victim. When we accept Christ as Lord, God dismisses all charges against sinners. We make an exchange: *our sin for His righteousness; our shame for His purity.* The Bible states,

Anyone who belongs to Christ has become a new person. The old life is gone; a new life has begun! ... For God made Christ, who never sinned, to be the offering for our sin, so that we could be made right with God through Christ (2 Cor. 5:17; 21) ... For we are God's masterpiece. He has created us anew in Christ Jesus, so we can do the things he planned for us long ago (Ephesians 2:10).

You say, "Who am I to be brilliant, talented, beautiful and wonderful?" God says, "Who are you *not* to be? You're my image-bearer!" Are you hindering God's work by not believing that you are *new, clean, pure, a masterpiece and righteous?*

9

SEXUAL SHAME OFF YOU!

Getting drunk allowed me (Kimberly) to act out the part of the seductress. The low self-esteem and mounds of shame disappeared for a while. I must have been a great actress because lots of guys wanted to have sex with me and I let them do what they wanted, regardless of whether I was attracted to them or not. I rejoiced in the attention.

One night I went to a party and got loaded (big surprise!). I met a great looking guy who lured me into one of the bedrooms. We had consensual sex. Then his girlfriend showed up and I became invisible. I continued to party-on to cover my humiliation and shame. The dude who hosted the party arranged for his friend to drive me home because I was so wasted. This stranger took me up to my apartment and I passed out. In the morning, I woke up naked and realized we had sex. He left a note with a phone number.

I didn't remember one thing about this guy, a guy who basically raped me. Yet I called the phone number because I desperately wanted to be in a relationship. The answering machine belted out a horrible, heavy metal, demonic-like song so, I hung up. I guess I had a little bit of dignity left ... or fear. Then ...surprise! One-month later I discovered I was pregnant. I didn't know which one of these guys planted the seed. *More sexual shame!*

Our sexuality is integral to who we are as individuals. Therefore, trauma of a sexual nature is a violation against our core self. My stories demonstrate the incredible damage created by sexual abuse and abandonment, and the resulting shame that leads to high risk behaviors.

It often starts because *every woman wants to know that beyond the sex—he loves her, needs her, and wants her, all the time.* (Compare to a man who wants sex because he "needs it" and wants to gratify himself.)

It's interesting that women like me get into relationships like this because we want not only want to be loved but saved. *If I can just find a great guy, then through him the hurts from the old relationships will vanish and I'll be fixed.* I finally learned that no relationship will save me. Only Jesus can do that. He and I have to do the healing work together.

The Silence

There are so many people in our world who are sexually wounded. Everyone has that one chapter they don't read out loud. Sadly, this world has created manipulators and exploiters who know how to masterfully use the female body for their own selfish interests. *Up to 40% of all women in the U.S. were sexually abused in childhood.* These numbers are high!

Dr. Michelle Stevens wrote,

> Sadly, we're so uncomfortable with the topic that we've banned it from conversation. The problem is: If we don't speak about childhood sexual abuse, how can we ever hope to make things better? If we want to protect children, thwart perpetrators, and help adult victims, we need to talk openly and honestly about the problem. ... But victims rarely talk about their shameful ordeals, creating a vacuum of information that leads to a lot of misunderstanding, insensitivity, and ignorance.[99]

Would it surprise you to know that Christians in New Testament times lived in a culture much like ours today? Men participated naked in the Olympic Games. Corinth had a temple with more than 10,000 cult prostitutes. Pornographic sexual positions were revealed beneath volcanic ash of Mount Vesuvius. The Greeks had a proverb, "women are for breeding, but boys are for pleasure."[100]

In the book of Genesis, chapter 19 openly talks of an attempted homosexual gang rape, as well as incestuous relations between a father and daughters. God later describes a horrible rape scene in chapter 34 and talks of more incest in chapter 35. Chapter 38 is about a man's one-night stand with his daughter-in-law. Amos 2:7 speaks of a father and son sexually using the same woman. God chose a sexually promiscuous woman, Rahab, to be one of Jesus's ancestors!

God is not prudish in discussing sexual sin. We need to remember that the human body and sexual intercourse were beautifully designed by God. It is *not* dirty or evil. Satan has done a marvelous job at messing up such a beautiful gift. God includes disgraceful sexual details in the Bible because these were real things that real people did—and they were considered sinful. They are just as relevant for us today. (Read Leviticus 18:6-30.)

Secondly, God designed our bodies to be a boundary. Dr. Henry Cloud wrote, "To invade another person's body, to cross over this person's boundaries, is the most basic act of abuse.

Sexual abuse is one of the most blatant examples of crossing boundaries, for someone takes what is not theirs. Our sexual functioning was meant to be freely shared with a partner of our own choice, not stolen against our will."[101]

If you were sexually abused, used, or assaulted, you probably suffer excruciating shame (among other strong emotions). The shame of any sexual violation to our bodies is the worst because our internal organs and our very soul is invaded; we lose a critical sense of having power and control over ourselves.

No matter how many times we heard the words "It's not your fault," we still blamed ourselves in some way—for being submissive; for not telling someone and allowing the sexual abuse to continue; for "enticing" the abuser with our behavior or dress; or because we felt some physical pleasure.

Many of us struggle with the pain of shame which comes out of both sexual abuse and sexual promiscuity. It has been found that a lifestyle of having sex with multiple partners can become a setup for abusive relationships. And vice-versa: A sexually abused kid often finds herself living a promiscuous lifestyle. A woman who has sex with a guy because she is seeking love, signs an emotional contract with him that can slowly turn abusive.[102] The terms: My body for your false love. Lisa Bevere wrote,

> It is very difficult for sexually broken or violated women to stand strong in the face of temptation. They have a hard time saying no even when they want to. They are overwhelmed with either lust or guilt, often both. They become victims and a magnet for sexual abuse and promiscuity.[103]

✝ When a female is treated as a sexual object, or presents herself as one, the woman made in the image of God remains hidden. In what ways do you relate?

An Abyss of Shame

"NO" is the source of sexual power; "NO" is the password to sexual peace. Women today need encouragement and permission to say "NO."
—"None of the Diseases"

Liz engaged in random promiscuous and extramarital affairs with men she met either at work or online. (This began after the death of her father.) Most were relationships she totally controlled—first by initiating them; later by ending them. She found the "sex game" exciting. Although she controlled these relationships, she never found them sexually satisfying. Nor was she sexually responsive to her husband. She admitted she used sex to "equalize" relationships, to stay in control. "It's safer this way" she believed.

For as long as Liz could remember, her mother had been hypercritical and constantly accused her of being "bad." She insisted Liz go to church and make an alter in her bedroom to ask for forgiveness. Liz felt closer to her father, a passive and quiet man, dominated by Mom. But as she entered puberty, Dad became more distant.

Liz's mom labeled her a "tramp" and "slut" even though she had no sexual experience. Liz chose to go to therapy and began recalling traumatic childhood events. She remembered severe beatings by her mom; mom inflicted vaginal douches and enemas, and then fondled her in order to "clean" her vagina. These rituals started when Liz was 8-years-old and ended at puberty. Believing she was worthless object, she began fantasizing she was different women—each one successful, beautiful, and in control.

By 13-years-old, Liz learned she had something every guy wants. She figured out if she became sexual with a guy, he'd give her some kind of emotional validation and sense of worth that she was so desperate for. *(Every female is in a power position.)*

At the core of Liz's being, she was ashamed; afraid of love, emotional attachment, and sex. In her search, she used men and then fled from the relationship. Coming to accept who she had become was difficult for Liz. Equally difficult was coming to accept that she had been forgiven by God. What she didn't know was that in His eyes, she was always just perfect.

Being used is often the mentality of victims, so they say they don't care, having lost something that was once priceless to them. In turn, they will use others, hoping to feel different, but always coming away feeling empty. They end up retreating into a dark abyss of shame.

What hooks us as women are the feelings of being loved, wanted, adored, and valued—which can be a kind of relational cocaine. We can get to the point that we can't turn down sexual offers and advances, even when we know in the end, we'll feel used and hate ourselves.

What happens is, we think of a past sexual encounter or relationship as history. We stuffed the memory down *but* the toxic residue remains and surfaces as insecurities and fears. It condemns and mutates into a desire to please: *I'll be any kind of woman you want me to be!*

When I look back all of my encounters, if I ask myself, "Which of those guys treated you well, and did you know what it felt like to be cared for?" The answer would be "none" and "no."

If you were sexually abused at an early age, how you view sex has been altered. Instead of the loving bond between a man and a woman that we've been designed for, that physical union becomes marred with painful memories.

How an individual reacts and copes to being exposed to a sexual relationship before they were mature enough to understand and handle it will vary from person to person. Having been violated, often repeatedly against their will, teaches a child that sex is not about love; it is about being used and treated as an object. Sex no longer holds the value it should; it simply becomes the means to an end.

When a person is taught a perverted version of sex, they bring that into other relationships. For example, Amber's boyfriend beat her up then expected sex. So, in Amber's following relationships she said she couldn't have a fulfilling sexual experience if she wasn't being hurt.

Other women gravitate to pornography. It's not just a man's problem anymore. More and more women are becoming addicted—and shamed. Studies state that 30% of porn addicts are female. When God tells us that He made us in His image, He is saying He values the femininity that comes from His very being.

† Describe again what kind of thoughts and emotions have been aroused in you.

Sexual Abuse and Dishonor

In a guy's arms, a woman feels so powerfully wanted, like someone is waving a magic wand for a moment over her insecurities, and then they evaporate.
—Paula Rinehart, Sex and the Soul of a Woman

Every month magazines such as Cosmopolitan, Seventeen, Marie Claire, and Glamour include topics such as *"How to Have Better Sex,"*

"How to Look Sexier," and *"How to Become a Sex Goddess."* Television industry statistics state that sex scenes have nearly doubled since 1998 and 70% of programming includes some type of sexual content. On average, these programs have five sexual images or scenes per hour! The objectification and exploitation of women is increasingly prevalent in online games and video games. Women are sex objects or victims of sexual abuse.[104]

This so-called sexual revolution has been a big part of my world, and I want to ask, "Can we please tell the truth; tell the real story?" This illusion that a man and woman can join their bodies intimately without changing the soul is crazy.

Don't women realize that every time their bodies are sexually dishonored that they lose a piece of themselves? Does she connect the feeling of numbness, as though her body is disconnected from the rest of her, to sex outside of its intended purpose?

My sexual wounds proclaimed, "I've lost so much of my self-respect and dignity, but I'm afraid of losing the guy. I have to give him my body." I remember not liking to be touched, while at the same time, engaging in sexual activity. I was seeking out my genuine needs—to be cared for, loved, and be close. Sex-only relationships depersonalize sex, making it impossible to engage in personal closeness. Intimacy involves trust, which may feel too threatening for either person to risk.

Sexual abuse survivors, including the promiscuous, experience the strongest, most toxic and destructive feelings of shame. Sexual abuse has an exceptional negative effect on a person. Since our sexuality is the most intimate part of a person, when there's inappropriate sexual contact or exposure, the result is *deep shame*.

Add to that, people in our lives who minimize or reject the abuse experience, and you have secondary and tertiary wounding. It was 13-years *after* confessing to having an eating disorder, abortion, and alcoholism that I publicly disclosed my sexual abuse and promiscuity history. That's how deep my sexual shame ran. It was the one chapter I didn't want to read out loud. Dr. Stephen Tracy wrote,

> God made our sexuality, particularly our genitals, very sensitive and personal and thus, susceptible to creating great shame. Our genitals are not shameful but are so intimate that any inappropriate exposure or contact can bring overwhelming levels of shame regardless of whether or not we chose to expose our bodies or consented to sexual contact.[105]

Holocaust survivor, Corrie Ten Boon, when asked what the worst thing she had suffered in the German concentration camps was, she responded, "It was the nakedness, so often having to be naked before all those jeering soldiers. That was the worst of all!" Once hanging naked on a cross for the public's view, Jesus identified with Corrie, just as He identifies with you, and your shame of being exposed.

Never forget, your power to fight off sexual sin is to launch an offensive attack against it—*power which comes from Jesus!* God says, "You've been designed by me to be loved, and valued, and cherished for the rest of your life by a man who beams when you come into a room. Strength and respect are your birthright!"

† Name the lies you believed. (I fell for the one that said if I could just establish a sexual connection with the guy I'm attracted to, then he'll be mine and we'll live happily ever after.)

Renewed Virginity

> *Whether we enter into it voluntarily or have it forced upon us, sexual sin causes severe wounds and scars that need more than forgiveness. They require healing.*
>
> –Barbara Wilson, The Invisible Bond

Sex, as designed by God, has been designed to be beautiful and transforming. Why then does it tear the soul apart? Answer: God's sexual boundaries have been dishonored. The most basic sexual boundary we know is that a parent, or any family member, is to not have sex, or make sexual propositions, toward their child. That's called incest.

When it comes to sex, common responses to sexual abuse/assault are being afraid of or avoiding sex; having difficulty becoming aroused; feeling emotionally distant; experiencing intrusive or disturbing images. If we are in a marriage relationship and sexual intimacy is a problem, one thing we can do is *encourage experimentation.* This means we tell our partner honestly we're not comfortable having sex, but would like to enjoy an intimate encounter with healthy physical touch.

You can feel the freedom to go only where you feel safe, and no further. If you do not feel pressure to rush the process, you may be surprised to find how quickly you do start to desire the very activities from which you feel threatened.

Sex Outside of Marriage

Another boundary breaker is sex outside of marriage. It's not the blueprint God created. God knows when this occurs there's a disturbing tendency to drift in the direction of power and manipulation. There is no pledge of love; no special meaning; no foundation to build lasting love and respect. The relationship caves in under the weight of selfishness.

Are you afraid that you had messed up so badly that God could never bless you, even worse, forgive you? The question we ask is: *Is it possible to have a genuine fresh start?* The answer is yes.

There is a concept called "renewed virginity"—an inner spiritual cleansing that brings wholeness and life. We cannot heal or grow when we are living in shame. The only force that can set us free and renew our spiritual virginity is the power of God. We are all sinners in desperate need of God's saving grace and forgiveness. Being a giver, forgiveness is His gift to us when we come to Him with a broken contrite heart. It begins with confession; with taking responsibility for what we recognize is sin.

The Bible says, *"If we confess our sins, he is faithful and just and will forgive us our sins and purify us from all unrighteousness"* (1 John 1:9). To *confess* is to admit to what we've done. We agree with God that our actions were wrong (versus trying to hide our sin). For those who confess, God promises He will *not* remember their sin. I know it's hard for us to forget, but if God can forget our past sins, then the least we can do is give ourselves a measure of grace and mercy each day. I also recommending reviewing the section *Exposing and Obliterating Our Shame* in "Shame off You." Pray:

> *Father, Deliver me from the seduction of sin and the need to satisfy my desires with the make-believe, rather than quench my thirst with You. Give me an untainted mind, a pure heart, and a deep desire to be pleasing in Your sight. By grace, help me to live a life that can be admired by my children, family, and myself. Amen.*

Breaking the Sexual Bonds

"I want to put up a sign that says, "Closed for repairs." –Tyra, survivor

#MeToo. Since October 2017, these two simple words have sparked an expanding movement that caught worldwide attention. Survivors of sexual assault are breaking the silence that has bound them with shame. They're broadcasting the secrets that up to now have protected the perpetrators. What the long-term effects of the #MeToo movement will be is unknown. However, there's a good chance it may become less stigmatizing for those who have survived sexual abuse and assault.

We heal when we *talk about sexual feelings.* As long as they remain hidden, they become shameful secrets. I don't want to present this task simplistically because it's not simple. It's hard to share them.

Sexuality is a highly charged subject for many. It's common to cover it up with pretense or jokes. It may be easiest to begin by sharing your feelings with a best friend or counselor. It's very helpful to share with other survivors. You'll find they too have similar feelings.

The best thing to do with your feelings is *feel them*. They are not the same as behavior. Sexual feelings, even arousal, doesn't have to lead to sexual activity. You don't have to act on the feelings unless you choose to do so. Learning to acknowledge them, and even enjoy them allows you to stop being a victim.

God created sexual feelings to be felt. Therefore, there is no harm in feeling them. *You* are in charge of when you will be sexual. This can be tremendously liberating. You are free to take charge of your life, to discover healthy relationships where you experience what it is like to touch and be touched in shameful sexual ways. You have the right to state clearly when you want to be touched, and how. You have absolute control over your body; nobody else.

Change Your Shame-Talk—Change Your Reality

I (Kimberly) wanted to free myself from the shaming belief that I was garbage because of my promiscuity. I invited Jesus, my therapist, to be part of my *Change My Self-Talk—Change My Reality* exercise. After reading my dialogue, write down your predominant judgement statement about yourself, then create your own dialogue with Jesus. Pray first.

When you do the exercise, you will come to separate and throw out the shaming labels and voices. You will separate them from who you are: a *new creation in Christ; not your past, nor are you sin!* Let God give you a new set of eyes to see yourself as you truly are—righteous, pure, and perfect. This is spiritual virginity!

1—Write down your judgement statement about yourself. *Belief*: I've slept with many men whose only motive was to use me, therefore, I'm an awful person. I'm garbage.

2—When I believe this thought, how do I react (the impact)? Since I feel dirty and unattractive, this thought makes me try to clean myself up with new clothes, makeup, dieting, and exercise. The shaming thoughts make me feel like an outcast, therefore I get drunk

Dancing in the Sonshine | 165

so I can morph into the man-pleasing seductress. I act contrary to the way God designed me. I fear asking, "Will you still like or love me if you know my secrets?"

3—How might I, and my life, be different without this thought? Without this thought I'd be free to be myself, the woman God created me to be; to engage in healthy relationships with men and other people.

4—Question and investigate the truth of the thought. Is it true? Yes.

> *Me:* If I weren't "garbage" these guys wouldn't have taken advantage of me. They would have wanted to pursue me as a girlfriend and not a sex object.
>
> *Jesus: Are you absolutely certain this is true?* (Look for the proof and inquire deeper.)
>
> *Me:* No. These guys never actually said, "I'm going to use you and don't desire a relationship with you." But, their actions said this.
> *Jesus:* What did their actions say?
>
> *Me:* "I'm going to coerce you into having sex with me. Then I'm going to leave and never contact you again unless I can coerce you into having sex with me again."
>
> *Jesus:* Why did you go along with them?
>
> *Me:* I wanted to be loved and desired.
>
> *Jesus:* The truth is these guys coerced and deceived you in a worldly evil act. You were looking for love, which is what I created you to seek because I am love. So, Kimberly, in this scene, who is clean? Who is unclean?
>
> *Me:* I was clean and they were unclean.
> *Jesus: "You are more valuable"* (Matthew 10:31).

5—Create a new belief; a new and truthful thinking track. The Bible says, *"Those who look to him [God] for help will be radiant with joy; no shadow of shame will darken their faces"* (Psalm 34:5). And Jesus said, *"you are more valuable"* (Matthew 10:31).

I'm not contaminated, dirty, or polluted, even though I encountered an unclean person. I'm clean and valuable and radiant! *He is unclean—not me!* Jesus will deal with him, and all the others who took advantage of me. No shadow of shame will darken my joy!

I finally realized that my inability to say no to a guy's sexual advances was due to fear and a deep need for love. I wasn't a whore. I was just seeking my God-given need to feel loved and accepted. I didn't have to feel guilty any longer. I had no more reasons to hate myself.

Alone Time with Your Therapist Jesus

The power of God—which is available to you—is the only force which can set you entirely free. Ephesians 1:19-20 says, *"I pray that you will understand the incredible greatness of* **God's power for us who believe him.** *This is the same mighty power that raised Christ from the dead ..."*

I suggest putting several hours aside one day to focus on breaking these sexual bondages. Find a place and time where you will not be disrupted. Some people like to fast. They find it helps them focus more intensely on God. Bring your Bible, paper, pen/pencil to the table. Turn the phone completely off. When you're finished, you may want to share your experience and emotions with a trusted friend. Ask her to pray with you.

I recommend beginning with meditating on and singing a couple of worship songs. You may then choose to praise God with a heart-felt prayer of gratitude and/or by reading Scripture that praises Him. Then begin bringing your past in prayer to God. Do not fear Him. He will not meet you with condemnation. Condemnation comes from the devil, other people, even ourselves—but never from God—*never!* It's not His heart.

One way to communicate with Him and enhance healing is through writing. Here are suggested subjects to write on:

- What your experiences with men and/or a sexual offender have led you to believe about yourself.
- How you feel about men in general; or certain types of men.
- About each of the men you've had a significant relationship with.
- About the flings, one-night stands; the friends with benefits: What was the negative emotional and spiritual impact?

A bondage-breaking healing exercise I did was to make a list of all the guys I had sex with (that I remembered). Many didn't have names; just a label. This took me almost a week to compile since I was covering a 17-year period (and even today another encounter may pop up into my memory bank). Then I expressed my feelings to God.

I confessed every single name or label and asked Him to forgive me for defiling my body. I asked Him to break every dirty shameful sexual bond tied to my soul. Then I proceeded to burn the list in the fireplace. The next day I shared the process with a safe friend who just loved me.

Paula Rinehart wrote, "When God comes into the center of our shame, he accomplishes the great exchange. He takes all our ugliness *on himself*, and he *gives us his beauty* in return."

No One Messes with God's Workmanship

In 1943, Rosa Parks (called the "Mother of the Civil Rights Movement") boarded a bus in Montgomery, Alabama. If you were black like Rosa, you entered the front door, paid the fare, exited the front door, and then had to reenter the bus through the back door, the accepted entrance for the "colored." On this one day, Rosa paid her fare but didn't reenter in the back. She walked down the aisle and took a seat. The bus driver, James Blake, refused to drive the bus until she properly exited and reentered the bus in the rear. After Rosa exited, he drove off and left her.

Twelve years later, the same bus driver, was driving a bus Rosa got on (she didn't know it at the time). She paid her fare and sat in an empty seat in the first row of black seats in the "colored" section. As the bus traveled its route, all the white-only seats filled up. Blake noticed a few white men were standing. He then moved the "colored" section sign behind Rosa and demanded that she and three others give up their seats to the whites.

In her biography, *My Story,* Rosa recalled, "When that white driver stepped toward us, when he waved his hand and ordered us up and out of our seats, I felt a determination cover my body like a quilt on a winter night. When he saw me still sitting, he asked if I was going to stand up, and I said, "No, I'm not." He said, "if you don't stand up, I'm going to have to call the police and have you arrested." I said, "You may do that." She was arrested and fined $14 but never paid the fine.

Her act became the symbol for a bus boycott led by the Rev. Dr. Martin Luther King Jr. and the Rev. Ralph D. Abernathy. Rosa Parks learned hard lessons in oppression but refused to be placed as "less than." She refused to be treated, in her own words, as a "second class citizen." By refusing her label, she showed others that they never have to accept "less than;" that they always have a choice.

What Rosa teaches us is: *No one can ever strip the image of God away from within us—no one can take our dignity away. No one—no one—can mess with God's workmanship!* Rosa taught "that people should stand up for rights, just as the children of Israel stood up to the Pharaoh."[106] She said, "I knew that He was with me, and only He could get me through the next step." It isn't enough just to pray. Sometimes trusting God means taking action too.

Actor Michael J. Fox said in *Saving Milly,* "One's dignity may be assaulted, vandalized and cruelly mocked, but it cannot be taken away unless it's surrendered."

Dancing in the Sonshine | 169

10

THE POWER OF CHANGED BELIEFS

Congratulations on making it this far. Some of the things you've read and processed through have been painful. They're painful because they reveal, perhaps for the first time, the depth of the suffering that goes with life's ugly circumstances. Other things are painful because they expose the truth—reality from God's point of view.

You are already a victor! No doubt you've already experienced God healing parts of your wounded heart and soul. Keep going. The angels in heaven are cheering you on!

Being Well-Deceived

The heart is deceitful above all things and beyond cure. Who can understand it?
—God, speaking in Jeremiah 17:9-10

One day on a subway train, a woman stood up, slapped the face of the man next to her, and then ran to the exit. Each of the passengers who saw what happened reacted in a personal way (called attunement).

A middle-aged man felt sadness for the man who was slapped. A younger woman was frightened. A teenage boy was stirred up. Another woman felt excitement. How could the same event trigger such a range of varying emotions? The answer is found in our mind's unconscious belief system.

- The sad middle-aged man thought, "He'll never get her back."
- The fearful woman thought, "She's going to really pay for that."
- The stirred-up teenager thought, "She humiliated him; like most women, she must be a real jerk."
- The excited woman thought, "Serves him right. She's strong!"

In each person's case, this event was interpreted, judged, and labeled instantly. The person's unique belief resulted in a different, distinctive, and personal experience of "truth" (which is why so many eye witness accounts are wrong).

William Hazlitt said, "Life is the art of being well-deceived." Experts say the inclination for self-delusion appears to be weaved into our genetic codes. Have you noticed that we simply believe that our judgment is better than the other guy's? We want to believe we have control over our lives, and self-delusion is usually required.

This is what Jesus meant when He said, *"For they look, but they don't really see. They hear, but they don't really listen or understand"* (Matthew 13:13).

The mind is powerful—but also easy to manipulate and deceive. That is what the advertising industry banks on … and why Satan targets our minds. Think about this: If a little girl has never seen a goat; never seen a picture or had one described to her, and you show her a cow and tell her it is a goat, she'll believe you. *We have no way to distinguish what is in fact really true.*

Adolph Hitler proclaimed, "If you tell a big enough lie and tell it frequently enough, it will be believed." Truth is *not* what is merely understandable, or what the majority says is true, or what makes us feel good. *Bondage always begins with a lie, even a half-truth.*

When a group of researchers evaluated decades of studies that measured how well people could distinguish truths from lies, they found that people's ability to spot deception was only a few percentage points better than a random coin flip.[107] In other words, it's hard to tell when people are misleading you and when they're not.

Do you remember the television program *The Newlywed Game?* We saw that getting to know someone quite often creates *an illusion* instead of reality-based insight.

Self-delusion enables us to protect ourselves. The child or wife who is being abused can believe, "This person loves me. This [violent behavior] is how he shows me." We are blind to just how much we've been influenced by other people and circumstances.

Growing up, we accept what we're taught without questioning. The rational, logical left brain convinces us that our thoughts, beliefs, and memories are true. We then rely on feelings generated from these beliefs, which are often false. If it *feels* right, it must be right. This is our emotional right brain at work. It's our default setting. It doesn't tell us that *feelings can lie!* No wonder the Bible says, *"Do not be deceived"* (Galatians 6:7).

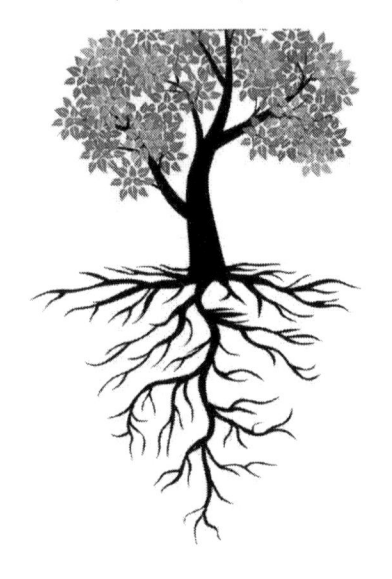

Life is like a tree, and our belief system is the massive root structure. Whatever our circumstances, we see everything that's going on through our personal "tree root" which creates and shapes our perceptions and beliefs, which in turn influences what we feel, what we say and do in the present. Thus, we create a future like our past.

Sadly, for most of us our tree roots are based on falsehoods. And nothing is going to change *until* a force—God—enters our lives and frees our minds from untruths. He can enable us to begin to see and "root out" false narratives through His pure and true lens.

A pill won't do did; only hard work. We begin by asking the Holy Spirit to intervene and pull out the roots. We tell Him we desire to reject untruths and create a new mind, a new set of values—a new life—untainted by any lies.

"I pray that the perception of my mind may be enlightened ... (Ephesian 1:18; HCSB); *"May the words from my mouth, and the thoughts from my heart be acceptable to you, O Lord, my rock and defender"* (Psalm 19:14).

With the power of God directing our minds, we can begin to recognize and eliminate the lies and control our thought life. Get into the habit of asking, *"Is there (biblical) truth to support my belief?"*

✝ How does it make you feel to know you've been deceived in many things?

Toxic versus Truth-filled Thinking

Whatever we excuse in ourselves that God does not excuse, we have deceived ourselves. – Diane Langberg, PhD

Apparently, women speak about 25,000 words a day; a man speaks about 10,000. There's an explanation: One man said, "My wife and I had words, but I didn't get to use mine."

Seriously, experts believe human beings process more than 50 experiences per second and have anywhere between 50,000 to 80,000 thoughts per day. That's an average of 2500 to 3500 thoughts per hour! Apparently, 98% of those thoughts are exactly the same thoughts from the day before; and *80% of them are negative … and false!* Scientists say the mind focuses on things other than what is actually happening in the present moment. In other words, our minds are extremely busy processing the wrong stuff.

There is a difference between a thought and a belief. A *thought* is something like, "I think I'll have a sandwich for lunch," or "This sweater doesn't match my pants." They tend to be fleeting and don't run our lives.

A *belief*, on the other hand, is more set-in stone; more black-and-white. We have our beliefs about God and Christianity, our identity, relationships, politics, etc. They tend to be judgments and run our lives—yet we're often not aware of them until it's time to examine them. Beliefs are more significant than thoughts.

We weren't born having negative beliefs about ourselves and other people. These evolved as we encountered people and situations that fed us negative, doubting, inhibiting messages and beliefs. Unaware, we swallowed these powerful toxins each day.

Scientists say positive emotions are fewer in number than negative emotions. Generally, we have a ratio of 3 to 4 negative emotions to one positive emotion.[108] Dr. Clifford Nass at Stanford University explains,

> The brain handles positive and negative information in different hemispheres. Negative emotions generally involve more thinking, and the information is processed more thoroughly than positive ones. Thus, we tend to ruminate more about unpleasant events.[109]

Science states that *75 to 98% of physical and behavioral illnesses come from a negative thought life.* Thoughts associated with a painful experience release negative chemicals that travel through the body changing the shape of the receptors on cells lining our hearts; thereby increasing susceptibility to illness. Toxic experiences cause brain cells to shrivel and die, compared to positive experiences which make brain cells expand.[110]

Numerous studies state that people who focused on negative aspects of themselves, or of life, generated waves of fear which released a flood of destructive neurochemicals into the brain.[111] Our bodies also release the hormone *cortisol* which weakens the immune system, kills brain cells, and causes weight gain. (Trauma *floods* the brain with cortisol.)

On the other hand, *75 to 98% of physical and behavioral healings come from a positive thought life.*[112] Our minds have the power of intellect, emotion, and free will, and, if empowered by the Holy Spirit, can change our thoughts. Consequently, we can make good choices that can positively change the body (including the brain), our feelings and behaviors—our lives.

Healthy, truth-based thinking today has become an integral aspect of treatment for everything from allergies to liver transplants. When we think positively instead of negatively, our tolerance for pain is higher, our recovery from illness and surgery is quicker, our blood pressure drops, our bodies release the hormone *DHEA,* and our brains release positive healthy chemicals.

✝ Would you say you can easily feel the impact of negative thinking and emotions in your mind and your body? Explain.

Intrusive Thoughts and Rumination

I am convinced that life is 10% what happens to me and 90% how I react to it. And so it is with you. Attitude is not everything, but it's almost everything. We are in charge of our attitudes. (Attitudes are our long-term memories composed of intertwined emotions.) –Unknown

Someone said, "Nothing in this world can torment you as much as your own thoughts." Byron Katie, author of *Loving What Is*, wrote "Behind every uncomfortable feeling, there's a thought that isn't true for us."

True or false: When you run into something troubling, your thinking runs through all kinds of scenarios.

How do you feel when someone criticizes you with (what you perceive to be) harsh words, sarcasm, ridicule or judgments? It may even be nonverbal; when someone gives you a look of disgust, disdain, even hatred. These actions are often at the root of "rumination."

Ruminate means we reflect on something *repeatedly* in our minds; we over-analyze; worry about a stressful event; we wrestle with the future. It's strongly related to depression and anxiety.

Could you say you are a "ruminator"?

Anxious people have a harder time suppressing negative thoughts, and thus, get caught up in the repetitive practice of rumination[113] —of chewing on a thought or a situation, just like a dog chews on a bone, always connecting the thought back to some perceived unchangeable and negative aspect. It's a recipe for depression and the blues.

This is because criticism lingers. We feel rejected. According to Chad Hall, Director of Coaching at Western Seminary, hearing criticism is not only painful in the moment, but it piles up and continues to do harm by keeping us in a stressful state.[114]

Every belief stored in our minds is our "reality"—our measure of truth. Just as the pain from one criticism begins to heal, a critical person opens the wound back up by firing another painful dart. Each new remark goes right onto the previous pile.

It's a fact: We carry around words of criticism and rejection for far longer than we do words of affirmation or encouragement. This is because our *personhood, our soul,* is attacked; compared with "feedback," which addresses our *behavior.* We carry around what I call "soul dirt."

This is what's going on in our brains: Following a painful act, toxic thoughts begin to form tracks in the brain. The tracks grow deeper and stronger every time we believe that another person has confirmed a particularly strong toxic thought: *That was really dumb of me.* We then feel even more *deficient, rejected, defeated, alienated, bad, unlovable,* and *unacceptable.*

For example, Sara's mom constantly tells her she isn't good enough. When her teacher tells her that her homework assignment didn't meet class standards, Sara repeats to herself *again* that she is not good enough, making that toxic thought track deeper and harder to get out of.

Critical words have a long life and remain toxic long after we think we've disposed of them. This is why we need God's Word, and honest and safe people in our lives—to speak truth and reality. Otherwise, we keep picking up those ugly remarks and ruminate on them unceasingly.

Fill in this sentence: "I tend to ruminate on something that bothers me [*75% or 50% or 25% or __%*] of the day.

The Spinning Top

Picture it: You've set sail. You're taking in the beauty of the ocean and the sky, reveling in the quietness. Then all of a sudden, a raging storm rolls in. Each wave threatens to overwhelm your boat. Then "He" rises from His sleep and rebukes the wind and the waves,

"Quiet! Be still!" (Mark 4:39). Can you hear it? Feel it? An instant calming at the hand of Jesus.

When I visualize the act of rumination, I see a spinning top. Did you ever have one of these as a kid? I did. I'd push repeatedly on the top and the cylinder would get spinning really fast. Then I'd thrust my hand down on the top and it would stop. "Be still!"

Our ruminating thoughts can start spinning out of control; spinning so fast that our minds become jumbled, which is because our brain circuitry has become muddled.

The opposite of rumination is *mindfulness*—focusing our attention on the present moment; a deliberate openness to connecting and taking in the presence of God. There are numerous instances in the Bible where we're told to "be still." In Hebrew the word "still" means to *cease striving; to collapse and fall limp*. Stop your mind's top and say, "In the name of Jesus, 'Quiet! Be still!'" Try it; it works.

Things Might Have Been Different ...

There is a way that seems right to a man, but in the end it leads to death.
—Proverbs 14:12

Are you one of the many women who've had a difficult and/or chaotic life, and consequently ruminate about how you'd have liked things to be different? *If only; I should have; I could have; Never; I can't.* Other words are: *would, ought* and *I wish I; I wish you had ...* Do these sound familiar: *it used to be... it could have been.*

Valerie's son became ill and she took him to the doctor, who diagnosed him with an ear infection. He got worse. Valerie took him to the Emergency Room. The doctor shared the same diagnosis. However, her son only got worse. She took him back to the ER where they diagnosed him with meningitis. Because his condition was so advanced, he died that day. Riddled with guilt, for months Valerie ruminated, "If only I ..." She judged herself as failing her child and began drinking to diminish the pain.

The truth was that she had no medical training. She took her son each time to physicians, who missed the diagnosis. She had fallen into the trap of judging herself on the outcome—rather than on her good actions and intentions as a mom.

When we feel we've lost control, it's easy to ruminate. All ruminating is good for is muddling our brain circuitry, re-wounding ourselves, stressing us out, leading to feelings of guilt, condemnation, depression, and other mental and physical disorders. These "strongholds of the mind" take us captive if we continue to feed and give power to the thoughts.

Mind transformation starts with thinking: *I'm willing to work at catching those thoughts and dealing with them, rather than entertaining them.*

Good news: 2 Timothy 2:7 tells us as Christians we have a *sound mind;* and 1 Corinthians 2:16 tells us we have the *mind of Christ.* This is powerful. It's also hard to comprehend because abusers are pros at invading our minds with confusion. Yet, God says *you have a divine mind!* You can do this!

It's been said that there's no such thing as a gray sky. The sky is always blue. However, sometimes gray clouds come out and cover up the blue sky. It's like that with our minds. We have the perfect mind of Christ yet it gets clouded with fearful patterns and distorted beliefs.

Gray clouds don't last; blue sky does. We've been designed by God to build good thoughts which lead to a healthy soul, mind, heart, and body, thereby, enabling us to receive God's love and good things for our lives—it's in our spiritual DNA! This means that you have the power to stop the stress of a disordered mind by investigating the thinking that lies behind it, and then change it.

† Elaborate on what it means to you to have "the mind of Christ."

Ruminating and Damaging Phrases

Learn to ask yourself this very important question, *"How can it be helpful and healthy to argue with or ruminate on something which has already happened or has not happened?"* Answer: It's not helpful.

Take the word *should*. How many times a day do you say or think, "I should …" or "My husband/boyfriend should …" or "That person should …" or "This organization should …"

When we create "should-thoughts," we are wanting reality to be different than it is. Let me also add, if you beat yourself up with a lot of *I should have* … statements, *please* tell yourself, "I was doing the best I could at the time."

These two phrases are popular: *You need to* … or *I want you to* … Much of our anxiety comes from living outside of our own business. When I start ruminating on the *You need to* … or *I want you to* … I'm in your business … and I need to get out. Your business is between you and God. When I'm in your business, then I'm not in my own, and I wonder why my life isn't working so well (a technique called "deflection").

I think there's a few exceptions: if you're a parent and are teaching your child responsibility; if someone in your life is doing something destructive which is affecting rest of the community and family, for example.

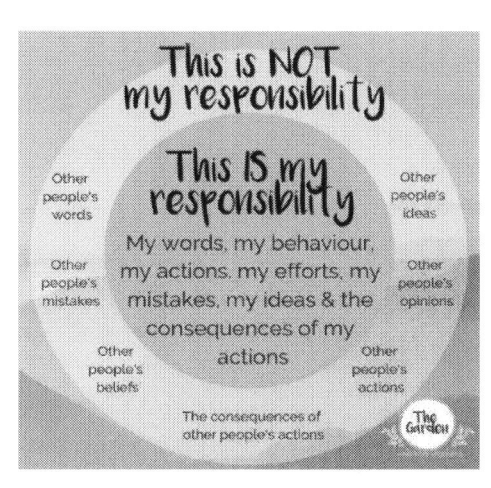

Peter said to Jesus, *"Lord, and what about this man?" Jesus said to him, "… What's that to you? You follow Me!"* (John 21:21-22).

Ask, "Whose business is it?" If it's not yours, then you have no reason to feel anxious. Simply put, to think that I know better than God what's best for someone is arrogance. And it only results in scrambled brain circuitry.

Dancing in the Sonshine | 179

Here's one last popular non-reality phrase: *I almost* … "I was *almost* a bride!" "I was *almost* hired."

How many *almost* moments have left you feeling devastated and unworthy, asking "What did I do wrong" and "What's wrong with me? Pay attention to how many times a day you think or say these popular words and phrases.

We need to get this: *Some, or much, of the stress we feel is usually caused by an expectation that is NOT reality!* We're either living in the past or future tense. Things in the past tense can't be changed; things in the future cannot be forecasted.

Instead we choose to focus on where we are—not where we wanted to be, or thought we should be, or wishing something hadn't been. That's not reality. Today counts. *We decide to accept "what is," fix our eyes on God, and leave the results to Him.* This is the best solution for overall health and well-being. It's our choice.

† Might there be any other negative phrases you use?

ATEs and PMSs (Thinking Errors)

One of the difficulties inherent in irrational thinking is it perpetuates itself.
– Albert Ellis, PhD

Why are you thinking these things? –Jesus, speaking in Mark 2:8

It's astounding how deceptive other people can be. Nevertheless, the biggest person who gets away with deceiving us is ourselves. We can choose to look for the truth or settle for untested perceptions. By settling for unverified perceptions, we refuse to consider other possibilities.

Let me ask you: *What if your thoughts aren't correct? What if they're not true?* Thoughts are not events, nor are they objective (means something most people agree upon). Thoughts are *subjective* (means my personal perceived reality;). Subjective thoughts run our lives.

Consequently, a huge number of women live with "Automatic Thinking Errors" (ATE) and have fatal PMS of the mind: "Powerful Mental Strongholds." We create them because we don't want to be blindsided by hurt, "punched in the gut" and caught off-guard. They're often a defense against shame.

ATEs and PMSs can become our master when we look to them to run our lives. Romans 6:1 asks a rhetorical question: *Don't you realize that you become the slave of whatever you choose to obey?*

Like a computer virus, it's not always easy to detect an ATE and PMS. False, infected, and painful beliefs are so engrained and have become *automatic* that we don't realize we have them.

Freedom from Unconscious ATEs and PMSs

Thinking patterns and beliefs will not change without new input. God wants to load a brand-new software program into your mind, one that He's designed specifically for you. We may not be able to control every single ATE|PMS from popping up, but with God's presence in our lives we can make good conscious choices. The greatest power God gives us is the power to change our minds. The Bible says,

> *Be transformed by the renewing of your mind* (Romans 12:2)
> *We take captive every thought to make it obedient to Christ* (2 Corinthians 10:5).

It can be very difficult to capture and renew something that's already captured us when we're not even aware of it. It may sound daunting to try to capture all of your thoughts and control your emotions. Yet when you begin to understand how you can do this, you will feel confident about change. Remember: *If God tells us to do something, He'll give us His power to do it.*

"Your mission, should you choose to accept it," is to become aware of, then quickly capture the deceptive thought; investigate it and then reframe it with truth. ("Reframe" means to think a different way about a behavior or experience; it is seeing things from a different angle.)

To "renew" means to "transform to new life"; to "take captive every thought" means we take responsibility for the thought and evaluate it in light of God's Word.

What thoughts do we have to capture? *Anything* that goes against God's truth—in other words, lies. The word "captive" has the meaning of confining or caging up.

"Quarantine" is a function of antivirus software that isolates infected files on a computer's hard drive. Take a moment and visualize taking an infected deceptive thought out of your mind, then quarantining it. Then we replace it with something good, like a thought of joy or gratitude, or a positive-self-affirmation like,

> *I am what I am today because of what I believed about myself yesterday. I'll be tomorrow what I believe about myself today—unless new positive experiences change how I think. My disordered mind can be turned into an ordered mind, and negative thought patterns broken!*

† Why might you be afraid to allow your thinking to be changed? (For example, fear of the unknown, conflict with family or friends?)

66/60

We all want to know, "How long will it take to see positive results?" Remember that thoughts are automatized into a habit through deliberate, repeated, and conscious thinking. When you repeat a pattern of behavior often enough, eventually you don't have to focus your attention on it anymore (the neural circuits underlying that behavior have stabilized in your brain, enabling you to respond to a similar situation automatically).[115]

Think back to when you learned to drive. At first every move you made was intentional—steering, braking, using the lights and wipers. Before you knew it, you drove automatically.

We now know the brain is not as rigid as once believed but is pliable and changeable. Our brains—young and old—have the ability to rewire and heal themselves when we learn and remember new things, called brain *plasticity* or *neuroplasticity* (*neuro* = brain cells; *plastic* = changed/altered. This is good news and bad news. Our brains change with *everything* we experience, both good or bad.

It will take, on the average 66 days to redesign our brains and form a new habitual thought pattern; and 60 days to break the old pattern.[116] God has given you a "sound mind" (2 Tim. 1:7, KJV). Neuroplasticity is His design for brain restoration and mind renewal.

Ask God to show you what issue you need to work on for the next 66 days. And remember the Antonio story. Don't expect to lift 100 pounds on your first visit to the gym. Most of us realize we won't meet our weight goals on the first, or second, even fifth visit. Certainly, we notice we're getting stronger each time we workout because we're exerting ourselves and growth is occurring. Like most things in life, this takes time and effort. So, give yourself a pep talk … and grace.

David prayed, *"With your help I can advance against a troop; with my God I can scale a wall"* (2 Samuel 22:30). Now you respond: *God, with your help I can … With You God, I will …*

Don't Crop the Image

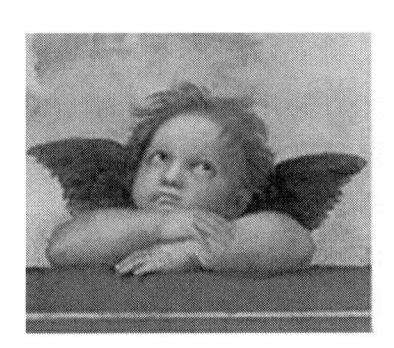

Take a moment to study this famous picture. No doubt you've seen it numerous times. This little cherub is quite famous in his own right. Heavily marketed, he has been featured in stamps, Christmas cards, postcards, T-shirts, lockets, mugs, wrapping paper and more.

What does this picture say to you or remind you of? What do you think is going on in this little cherub's mind?

Now take a look at this second picture. This is the original painting, known as "Cherubs from the Sistine Madonna" by Sanzio Raphael. The masterpiece was created in 1514. It is quite different from the first picture.

When viewing the original picture, the message becomes clearer. These two cherubs are looking up—up to heaven where God resides. The Catholics believe they are Saints Sixtus and Barbara, looking up to Mary.

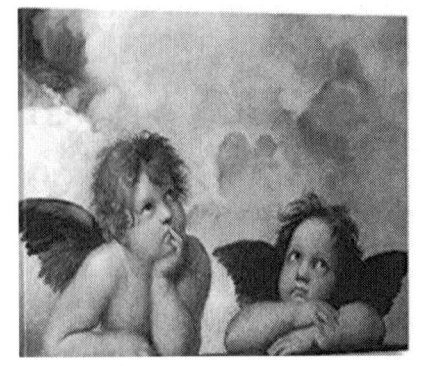

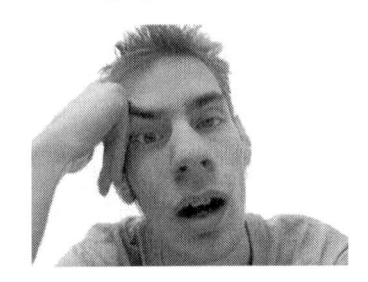

What's my point? We tend to "frame" ourselves, other people or situations with our limited view. We "crop" reality. For example, we may associate the image of the cherub in the cropped picture with our teenage son—the son who constantly whines that he's so bored at home. We judge what's going on in the cherub's mind based on our personal judgment of kids who look like this.

This is far from reality. In the cropped picture we don't see the background and history.

Tanya's struggles and fears as an adult go back to when her dad left her and her mom at age six. She vividly remembers him driving off, believing he didn't care.

She asked Jesus to bring all the information about this experience to her mind. She then had an image of the anguish that was on her dad's face as he drove away. A flood of understanding and relief filled her when she finally realized that leaving his daughter that day pained him greatly. This encouraged her to have a conversation with him about that day (she had refused to have anything to do with him since then). She learned about the ongoing conflicts between him and her mom, and how he felt leaving was something he had to do to benefit them both. She got a view of the full picture.

It's never a black and white issue. We forget we have a limited perspective. I challenge you not to put your own frame of perception and judgment around your story, and around other people and their stories. Let go of your limited view. As one writer brilliantly stated, "Judgement will always reduce the size of the frame."

We all do the same thing. We interpret, judge, and label a person/event instantly. Our unique belief results in "our" experience of truth which may be a complete 180 degrees from someone's else perspective.

11

SET YOURSELF FREE WITH FORGIVENESS

I started hanging out with the tough girls that I could relate to. They all had the same kinds of things going on in their homes—somebody was drinking or abusive, or they came from a broken home. We could relate because we were all angry and wanting to get even with the people who hurt us and the world. We fought anyone and everyone. We formed a gang called Satan's spades. The anger took over. I wanted to hurt people and kill everybody.
–Excerpt from *When God's Spirit Moves* by Jim Cymbala

For most of us, our wound is a result of something bad someone else has done to us. We may feel the need to retaliate in some manner; after all, "What happened to me is not right! The offender needs be held accountable and suffer for the pain he caused me!"

Or perhaps, you think the "Christian thing" to do is stuff the agony and 'forgive and forget.' Many abused women, in order to survive, try this tactic. But despite your resolve, the wound keeps breaking back open, you relive it, and the injustice and pain engulf your mind all over again. Your desire is to forget it, but the suppressed resentment just doesn't disappear. You ruminate and obsess over the wound.

The other thing is, nothing wreaks havoc on the body like bitterness, anger, resentment and hatred. When we hold onto these toxic emotions, the cells in our bodies are put into a tense state, which damages our immune system and impairs our ability to think and remember things clearly.

Contrarily, when we forgive, we let go of negativity and pain; thereby we restore our bodies and souls. The result: Healthier relationships, greater spiritual and psychological well-being; less anxiety, stress, and hostility; lower blood pressure; fewer symptoms of depression and cardiovascular disease; a lower risk of: substance abuse, cancer, hormonal changes, immune suppression, arthritis, and possibly impaired neurological function and memory.

Forgiveness: is giving up both resentment toward someone else, and the right to get even, no matter what that person has done. Unforgiveness, then, describes a deliberate refusal to let go of ill will or the desire for revenge, based on the attitude that the person has to pay for the offense.

It is not about getting our right to justice; that's God's job. It's about forgiving others as the Lord has forgiven us. This is what this chapter is all about. We can trust God to handle unfairness and give us the power to forgive.

Forgiving is *not* the same as "pardoning." Pardoning releases people from punishments or the consequences due them; forgiveness doesn't. It's important to recognize that forgiveness is not a "one and done" deal. *The deeper the wound, the longer the process.*

This is important: When it comes to the subjects of forgiveness and confrontation, abuse survivors attach very different meanings and emotions to these subjects. No two women will handle them quite the same. Yes, forgiving is a big part of healing, but many make it the goal of healing. They may be made to feel because they're a "Christian" they must forgive or else they'll make God mad—which may feel like more manipulation. Personal restoration is always the first step to healing; forgiving an abuser is second; and confrontation, third. If you haven't worked through the previous chapters—really done the work—forgiveness can feel premature which can make you feel revictimized.

The "F" Word

For many, the word *forgive* is the ultimate "F" word. Forgiving is *not* the same as "pardoning." Pardoning releases people from punishments or the consequences due them; forgiveness doesn't. Forgiveness seems so difficult because we make it about our feelings.

It is not a feeling. If it were, we would rarely forgive because we wouldn't "feel" like it. We choose to trust God to handle unfairness and give us peace and the power to forgive.

It is not about getting our right to justice; that's God's job. He is the avenger of all injustice—and fair. *"For the LORD loves justice, and he will never abandon the godly. He will keep them safe forever, but the children of the wicked will die" (Psalm 37:28).* Justice will come either today on earth or in the future in heaven, but rest assured, justice will prevail!

God insists we forgive because He has forgiven us (Colossians 3:3). Being a follower of Christ means forgiving others as He has forgiven us. We're expected to model and show the world a different picture of what revenge and retaliation mean. He wants us to show mercy to others because He's shown mercy to us.

An Act of Obedience and Self-Love

Forgiveness is not about the other person, and it's not only about obeying God's Word—it's an act of self-love. There are so many spiritual, emotional, physical and relational benefits we will receive.

When we choose to forgive, we let go of negativity and pain; thereby we restore our bodies and souls. The result: Healthier relationships, greater spiritual and psychological well-being; less anxiety, stress and hostility; lower blood pressure; fewer symptoms of depression and cardiovascular disease. Plus, a lower risk of: substance abuse, cancer, hormonal changes, immune suppression, arthritis, and possibly impaired neurological function and memory.

There are consequences if we don't forgive. Unforgiveness, and its associated emotions, gives Satan a foothold in our lives from which he is able to stir up anger and bitterness (Ephesians 4:26-27) and other toxic emotions. Despite our attempts to contain it, a bitter spirit comes out in our words and actions (Hebrews 12:15). It reaches its ugly tentacles into our thoughts, attitudes and into our bodily systems.

Worse, unforgiveness damages our fellowship with God. Jesus gave us a serious warning, *"If you do not forgive others, then your Father will not forgive your transgressions" (Matthew 6:15).* This doesn't mean we lose our salvation, but it creates a barrier in our relationship with God.

Bottom line: We can't be right with God and be at odds with someone else (1 John 2:9). I dislike clichés, but this simplistic one fits: *Let go and let God:* Let go (of the toxic emotions) and let God (radically change your heart and mind). For our sanity and health, and our relationship with God, we have to get our eyes off the offender and our right to get even, and onto Jesus.

The Perfect Judge

This teaching may feel disturbing, as if the offender is going to get away with the offense. *No transgression gets past an all-knowing God.* The Bible says God is the God of judgment and is a good and fair Judge. *"Do not take revenge, my dear friends, but leave room for God's wrath, for it is written: 'It is mine to avenge; I will repay,' says the Lord" (Romans 12:19; 2: 5-11; 2 Thess. 1:6-10).*

The Bible provides numerous promises that God will take care of the offenders.[117] In other words, He will take on the burden and pain for us. The cliché, "Let go and let God" applies here.

As someone said, "God doesn't need us to police the world." Therefore, we shouldn't waste precious energy and time nurturing a bitter root of anger or hate or retaliation. God's a better judge than we are and knows every person better than we do.

Cecil Murphy wrote, "Even if I knew why God hadn't intervened in my situation, would it make any difference? Would it make me feel better? It still happened. One day the perpetrators will have to stand before God for their sins."

Judging Favorably

In *The Passion of the Christ*, a film that broke box-office records, the audience witnesses an according-to-the-Bible account of Jesus's last hours on this earth. The film centers around His arrest, trial, torture, crucifixion, and resurrection, events commonly known as "the passion." If you saw this film, no doubt, like me, you were shaken up.

Jesus underwent a horrific torture and humiliation for our sins. What the movie didn't show was the horrendous details of an actual crucifixion. Crucifixion was one of the most disgraceful forms of death and most dreaded methods of execution in the ancient world. The method of crucifixion was so brutal that I refrain from describing it in detail. Let me just say Jesus was beaten horrifically and His body torn from head to toe. The soldiers far surpassed their orders in maliciously violating Jesus. To further shame the victims, the Roman soldiers nailed them to the cross naked. Yet, as Jesus hung nailed to the cross, He advocated something that stuns us, *"Father, forgive them. They don't know what they're doing" (Luke 23:34).*

Imagine having someone humiliate, ridicule, abandon, reject, and torture you, and then drive stakes into your hands. Would you feel like praying for them? No way! Scripture says, *"He did not retaliate when he was insulted, nor threaten revenge when he suffered. He left his case in the hands of God, who always judges fairly" (1 Peter 2:23).*

Human nature calls for revenge and retaliation. Not Jesus. He didn't yell from the cross, "You bad people, you're in big trouble now!" even though He had every reason to be righteously infuriated. Sinless, He did nothing to deserve crucifixion. These three important words, "Father, forgive them," modeled what He taught people about forgiveness and loving their enemies *(Luke 6:27-28).*

What has helped me immensely is to understand and the apply the concept of *judging favorably*. Jewish culture has emphasized the need to "judge favorably" for thousands of years. The rabbis declared that "judging others in favorable terms" is as important as visiting the sick, praying, or teaching the Scriptures to your children. If we ask God to help us see a situation differently, we can change our perceptions—we can judge favorably, just as 1 Samuel 16:7 states, *"The LORD doesn't see things the way you see them. People judge by outward appearance, but the LORD looks at the heart."*

Reframe the Offense

You never really understand a person until you consider things from his point of view . . . Until you climb inside of his skin and walk around in it. –Harper Lee

Jenna conveyed to her therapist, "I now realize the person who hurt me is a victim and suffering with his own pain. He didn't realize he caused me suffering because he was too blinded and wounded himself." This is called "reframing."

No healthy and functional person wakes up one day and decides to abuse or offend another person. *Broken hurt people hurt people; broken hurt people raise broken people.* It's never a black and white issue; we have a limited perspective. What we choose to forgive is the flawed human being who did a very bad thing (or things) as a consequence of their own wounding and flawed belief system.

Scripture says, "*For all have sinned and fall short of the glory of God. … There is no one righteous, not even one*"—including us *(Romans 3:10; 23)*.

The fact is: When someone is cruel, he or she is usually afraid. Many therapists agree that *shame-based fear*—the fear of never feeling noticed, of not feeling loved or of belonging, nor having a sense of purpose, is a large reason for an offender's bad and cruel behavior. Another reason is their belief system is all messed up.

It's remarkable how our attitude will change when we begin to bless and pray for those who've wounded us. We can lift them up to God and try to imagine what an awesome person they could be if they had a genuine relationship with Jesus. The Lord can so transform our hearts that instead of wishing evil upon them, we desire good for them. Have faith!

Many of my prayers to God have been, *"Help me change my mind and heart toward this person and help me to try to see [name] as you see [name]."*

Another benefit of reframing the event is we are adding a positive experience (memory) to the negative one, thereby diminishing its power to incapacitate us.

Ask God to reframe your belief about the person. What works for me sometimes is to try to see them as "sick" versus "bad." We don't tend to be so peeved at people who are sick. Or, as one therapist asks her clients, "What would your response be if the offender was your own child?"

† Describe how "judging favorably" feels to you at this moment.

This All Sounds Good, but How?

Then he fell on his knees and cried out, "Lord, do not hold this sin against them."
—Stephen, speaking in Acts 7:60

This is the question I'm always asked. In the book of Colossians, the apostle Paul talks about getting to the place of unselfishly caring for people. He used the phrase "love in the Spirit." This isn't an earth-based love; it's the Holy Spirit's love. Only He has the ability to replace our human limitations and carnal tendencies supernaturally.

"'Not by might nor by power, but by my Spirit,' says the LORD Almighty" (Zechariah 4:6). We have a great power available. Since we are created in His image, this means we *can* come to forgive.

"Love in the Spirit" is totally separate from human ability. This is a great reason to be connected to God each and every day, and pray for the "love in the Spirit" to invade our hearts and minds. It's a constant petition because as humans we tend to fail repeatedly at it; we're powerless (Romans 5:6).

When we start to let go of our convictions against the person and give them to God; even come to love the person, that's an indisputable sign of the power and activity of the Holy Spirit working in us. He specializes in changing our nature—a radical change in mind and heart and soul. *Only the love of God flowing through us can enable us to judge favorably, reframe and enable us to forgive the unforgiveable.*

Judging Yourself Favorably

Tara said, "When I was a kid, my dad did sexual things to me. He said all daddy's do these things to show their little girls they love them. For most of my youth and young adult life, I didn't feel I had to forgive him because I did something to attract him."

Have you noticed we are often more unforgiving towards ourselves than we are others? Do you struggle with forgiving yourself?

Self-blame is a common response to being abandoned or rejected or abused. We tend to assume responsibility for something that *happened to us*; yet, we did nothing wrong. No doubt, pain is the cause of our actions. Therefore, we need to reframe, reinterpret and apply the same principles about judging another person favorably to ourselves. Jesus sees us as forgiven and perfect, therefore we need to see ourselves with His set of eyes.

We do need to "pardon" ourselves for having behaved in ways that perhaps brought pain to others due to our pain, and make amends where necessary. John Bunyan said, *"No child of God sins to that degree as to make himself incapable of forgiveness."*

Champion Your Little Girl Hurt Self

The inner child represents our authentic self. When not nurtured, our hearts and minds close; we're unaware of our feelings and inhibited in our expression. Think of the little girl/young woman inside yourself who was abused and treated badly.

Imagine Jesus saying, "I see you Daughter back in that moment. You have My support, Love and care."

Connect with her as you would your own child or a best friend. Show her forgiveness and compassion, nurture and nourish her; have empathy for the girl/woman who has been grievously offended; champion her; get stirred up for what she had to experience. Finish this sentence, "What I want you to know is ..."

Write an impact letter. Tell the person the impact their actions had on your life. *Don't send it* unless you feel certain about doing so. Once it's sent, it's sent. Effective dialogue when challenging someone can go like:

- I feel …
- When you …
- What I would like …
- What I'm willing to do is …

Decisional and Emotional Forgiveness

Forgive—We are talking about choosing to do something that goes contrary to our feelings. Forgiveness seems so difficult because we make it about our feelings. It is not a feeling. If it were, we would rarely forgive because we wouldn't "feel" like it. We'll never get there.

We need to recognize that feelings take time to heal after the choice to forgive is made. There are two concepts of forgiveness we need to understand: *decisional* and *emotional*.

The *decisional forgiveness* process usually comes first. It's not a feeling but *an act of my will* to obey God. I won't necessarily feel love for the person, especially if the offense was great. I choose to judge favorably; not to hold this injustice against the person or seek revenge. I choose to put my faith in God's justice. I also remember that in my sin I betrayed God, yet He forgave me. Therefore, I need to forgive others.

Decisional forgiveness says, *I acknowledge the things you did (or did not do) that caused pain. I'm taking you off my hook and putting you on God's hook. I'm not going to let you and the unforgiveness hurt me and my relationship with anymore.*

Pray something like: *Father, I let go of the person who wounded me and the lie (name the lie). I choose to forgive (the person) for (name the offense) because it made me feel (share your emotion) I now choose to let go of the (name the emotion such as anger or bitterness or resentment). I ask You to heal my damaged emotions. Thank You for setting me free from the bondage of my pain. Now I ask You to release (offender) from his/her pain.*

This shows God we mean business. I believe God honors our *decision* to obey and forgive; we're "good" with Him once again.

Emotional forgiveness is the process of replacing negative feelings with positive emotions. With decisional forgiveness, I choose to forgive you, but I'm unable to manage my negative emotions. One of the greatest American writers, F. Scott Fitzgerald wrote, "There are open wounds, shrunk sometimes to the size of a pin prick, but wounds still." My heart needs time to catch up with my decision to forgive.

Decisional forgiveness takes place instantly and is based on Colossians 3:13: *"Forgive as the Lord forgave you."* On the other hand, emotional forgiveness can be a restoration process—a process of emotionally releasing and forgiving, time and again. As time goes on, we often recognize new losses. We need to re-forgive because our losses tend to accumulate. God understands how difficult is to emotionally forgive and is always ready to help us.

One last clarification—as a wounded person, there is no guarantee that you'll never return to older feelings. *This does not mean that you have not forgiven the person.* It is not uncommon to be triggered by something, and then strongly feel the rage. This is part of the natural fight/flight response; a healthy response to violation that is wired in us. For these complicated reasons it's vital to take your feelings immediately to Jesus and talk to a safe person.

(By the way: This two-step process also applies to intimate relationships, particularly marriage. Most of us will go through seasons when we don't particularly like our spouse. It is in these cases we must make the decision to be kind and loving, even if our emotions don't agree. Love is not only a verb; it also means taking action (see 1 John 4:16-19). Of course, if there are sinful offenses that need to be addressed, then those must be dealt with.)

We are able because God is able.

†††

Here's my motivation for forgiving: Actress Sara Miles once said, "An unforgiving nature reflects in your face. Holding negative energy drags down the facial muscles, puckers one's frown and causes lines around the mouth. Working daily on forgiveness is the cheapest, most effective facelift in the whole wide world." ☺

What Forgiveness is NOT

I forgive my family and abuser as it unhooks me, but forgiveness doesn't mean I welcome abusive people in my life. —Tara

There are many misconceptions about forgiveness and expectations of behavior. Understanding what *forgiveness is not* is often the key to making the decision to forgive, and therefore, setting ourselves free emotionally.

Forgiveness is Not Letting the Person off the Hook
Often an offender's actions destroy lives. This doesn't mean you don't hold the person accountable. King David committed adultery, then murdered a man in an effort to cover his sin. God judged David's sins and he paid dearly for the rest of his lifetime.

When God forgives us, He's not saying past behavior is disregarded. U.S. laws demand people be held criminally responsible for their crimes. Forgiveness involves mercy and grace, but it also involves accountability. If we let the person off the hook too easily, they may conclude the offense wasn't really that serious. God sets penalties, and He gives us the ability to do so.

Secondly, abusers are very good at getting us to take the blame for their wrongs. If you find yourself apologizing for how you caused the person to offend you or others, you've been significantly misguided and deceived. The mirror must be put up to their face. They must recognize and admit their wrong, then ask for forgiveness.

Forgiveness Does Not Excuse, Minimize or Justify

Janna's parents demanded she forgive her brother for making her watch pornographic movies with him. Janna agreed in order to keep the peace.

You may be asked to forgive because your family wants you to. Families have a way of justifying or minimizing what's taken place. Many offenders want you to take responsibility for their behavior. Forgiveness is not saying, "It's no big deal." If it's no big deal, there's nothing to forgive.

Forgiveness Does Not Forget

There is a word which cannot be associated with forgiveness: "forget" (as in "forgive and forget"). The fact is, we don't forget. Brain studies reveal whatever is significant to us is stashed away in our long-term memory.

Paul said he is, *"Forgetting what is behind and straining toward what is ahead"* (Philippians 3:13). The biblical word "forget" in this context doesn't mean "put out of one's mind." It has the *meaning of letting go— not allowing the past experiences to dominate the future.* We see this in the parable of the prodigal son (see Luke 15). The father didn't dwell on the son's past mistakes. His heart desired to take him back into the house and then celebrate his return.

We must understand God's reconciliation process: when we forgive, the offense is forgotten *as far as the relationship is concerned* because it's no longer relevant to the relationship. The memory isn't erased; the facts of the event aren't expunged. *We are choosing not to dwell on it anymore.*

Forgiveness Is Not Contact or a Future Relationship

Speaking of her adulterous husband, Lark said, "I know I'm supposed to forgive and trust, but I can't let myself be hurt again. If I let him back in, I know he'll hurt me again." Who said anything about letting him back in and trusting him? People are reluctant to forgive because they don't understand the difference between forgiveness and trust and reconciliation.

Forgiveness has to do with the past. The wounded person makes the choice to let the offense go. Trust and reconciliation have to do with the present and the future. *Forgiveness is not an expectation of a future relationship with the person.* No mere words can bring about a significant repair. *The offender must prove he/she's changed their behavior over time and are trustworthy.*

Lark finally realized she would relieve herself of the bitterness, resentment, and pain, if she chose to forgive her husband for adultery, even though she had biblical grounds for divorce. She also learned that by making the decision to forgive her husband, this didn't change him; it didn't make him any more trustworthy. Until he could prove he was, she chose to separate from him and move on. She chose to trust God to judge him fairly. She put boundaries into place so this event didn't happen again. They need time to take the steps required for true restoration, called *repentance*.

Repentance is from the Hebrew word *teshuva*, "to turn around or change direction or purpose." In Greek the word is *metanoia* which implies a heart or thought change. It's an inner change that leads to an outward change of lifestyle. Without repentance, sometimes a relationship cannot be restored.

The definition of "trust" is: *What is important to me is safe with you in this situation (or any situation)*. Conversely, "distrust" is: *What is important to me is NOT safe with you in this situation (or any situation)*. Trust is always earned. The person must prove to be faithful, honest, and have integrity. Therefore, it takes time to rebuild, and requires patience.

Research has shown that it can take up to 2-years to develop an authentic attachment bond when there *hasn't* been any type of wound or betrayal. Therefore, the person who is working to change and earn your trust must give you "all the time in the world" to trust again.

Warning: If you believe this person has a personality disorder or is or dangerous, do not meet with him/her. In my opinion, you'll most likely be dragged right back into the same old mind games. You can forgive them, but for your safety you don't have to tell them you forgive them. You are in this good place now because of your distance away from this person.

Forgiveness is Not Waiting for an Apology
Some say, "I'll forgive him as soon as he says he's sorry." There are people who will never apologize and never confess or admit their sin. Or they'll apologize, yet continue in their destructive, rebellious, and foolish behavior. Others will say, "Look, I apologized. Drop it!" This isn't a genuine apology; the person simply wants to get out of a predicament and silence the other person.

Many offenders typically demand you accept their apologies and forget the incident. This is an indicator of lack of repentance. They're saying they don't want to look at your wound or be accountable for what they did. Longing for a genuine apology from someone who has betrayed you is understandable, but frequently unrealistic. We need to let go of any expectation of getting the response we want.

In the long run, what matters is not whether the person "really meant it," what counts is there is genuine repentance and no repeat performance.

Forgiveness Does Not Stay Silent
The healing process for us, and the repentance process for the offender, requires talking about the offense. Healing evolves when we talk about the pain and have our feelings validated. When the person allows you to express your feelings, and they feel true sorrow, then it's possible to move forward and *"forget what's behind."*

Let me wrap this up by saying: People who commit serious harm can't be reached through conversations that, in their mind, further shames and blames them. You may need to reduce your expectations to zero if you are seeking some kind of remorse and repentance from the person.

People can't be honest with us if they can't be honest with themselves.

† Describe how this "Forgiveness is Not" list made you more receptive towards forgiveness and/or has help set you free from a certain person and/or situation.

Authentic Repentance

A relationship can begin the process of restoration when the offender shows signs of humility and authentic repentance. I love Bruce Wilkinson's description: *"Repentance means you change your mind so deeply that it changes you."*

This is not the same as remorse. When repentance is real, there is a groaning from the spirit that truly means, "I'm sorry. I don't ever want to do this again." As it states in Job 34:31-32, *"people say to God, 'I have sinned, but I will sin no more' Or 'I don't know what evil I have done—tell me. If I have done wrong, I will stop at once.'"* The person is willing to look at the truth.

Jesus told this parable called the Pharisee and the Tax Collector (See Luke 18:10-14). Scripture says,

> *One day Jesus told his disciples a story to illustrate their need for constant prayer and to show them that they must keep praying until the answer comes (v. 1) ... Then he told this story to some who boasted of their virtue and scorned everyone else." (v. 9).*
>
> *Two men went to the Temple to pray. One was a proud, self-righteous Pharisee, and the other a cheating tax collector. The proud Pharisee 'prayed' this prayer: 'Thank God, I am not a sinner like everyone else, especially like that tax collector over there! For I never cheat, I don't commit adultery, I go without food twice a week, and I give to God a tenth of everything I earn.' But the corrupt tax collector stood at a distance and dared not even lift his eyes to heaven as he prayed, but beat upon his chest in sorrow, exclaiming, "God, be merciful to me, a sinner." I tell you, this sinner, not the Pharisee, returned home forgiven! For the proud shall be humbled, but the humble shall be honored.*

Pharisees were regarded as the most devout religious group of men in Jesus's time. The name "Pharisee" comes from a root word that means "pure." These guys sought purity in *all* things. They were famous for their religious enthusiasm and piety (means a dutiful spirit of reverence for God). They believed they were morally superior to most other human beings. They had pride in themselves and disdain for others. In contrast, the tax collectors were at the opposite pole. They were despised. Certainly, a repentant tax collector defied all the stereotypes of the day.

The surprise of the parable doesn't lie in the Pharisee's prideful attitude, but in the tax collector's response. He cries for mercy and grace, recognizing his brokenness. Something brought him to that "hit rock bottom" or "come to Jesus" moment.

Toby is a good father, but has an erratic binge drinking problem. He goes on binges and becomes verbally and physically abusive to his wife and kids. After beating his wife one evening, their 12-year-old called 911 because her face was covered with blood. Toby was arrested for battery.

This event finally brought him to his senses. Toby saw the face of his wife and he cried like a baby, vowing to never be violent again. He admitted he needed God in his life to change him. The next week a friend took him to a Celebrate Recovery meeting. With God's help, his life—and his family's life—moved in a new direction. It is possible the tax collector had a similar experience—an event made him aware of how low he had gotten.

Luke 3:8 states, *"Prove by the way you live that you have repented of your sins and turned to God."* When someone is truly repentant, he or she will follow the process of the *Six R's to Authentic Change* (see Appendix E). They will admit that God is in control, and they will relinquish being the king or queen sitting on their own throne, and acknowledge Jesus is King over their life.

Now that you have completed this chapter, consider:
- How has your definition of forgiveness been reshaped?
- If you skipped this chapter, in what ways would it affect your growth and healing?

12

CHANGE YOUR MIND AND MEMORY— CHANGE YOUR REALITY

Adolph Hitler's body guard was often asked in interviews whether he heard Hitler speak of the Third Reich's murder of 6 million Jews. He always replied no. In 2005 he said, "If Hitler really did all the terrible things people said he did, how could he have been our Fuhrer?"[118] (Are you kidding me?) The evidence showed Hitler did horrendous things.

Paul wrote to the Colossian church, "*See to it that no one takes you captive through hollow and deceptive philosophy ...*" *(Colossians 2:8).* Why would Paul give us this advice? Because once we come to believe something is true, we give it up reluctantly, or not at all, like Hitler's body guard. Once a belief takes root in our mind, it becomes very difficult to dislodge. To give them up threatens our sense of self.

What if our thoughts aren't true? This is a strong probability. Therefore, we've got to examine them—those hollow and deceptive subjective philosophies—and remove the deceits. This sounds impossible, and it is, which is why we ask God to reveal them to us. He will.

You can choose to skip this work and leave your toxic thoughts and false beliefs in your unconscious (the most dangerous) or ask God to bring them into your conscious mind one thought at a time so you can *express it, interrogate it,* and then *remove it*—thereby, changing reality and your life.

God wants us to believe based on evidence, so get ready to inquire and investigate your thoughts, and set yourself free! *(John 8:36)* These reflective investigative exercises will enable you to take your toxic thoughts captive and not allow anyone to capture you with empty deceptive philosophies.

Cognitive Dissonance

Once you begin this process, no doubt, you will experience what is called in psychology "cognitive dissonance." This is when a very strong conviction or belief we have is met with what our minds believe is contradictory evidence.

The problem is that core beliefs act as a filter that only lets in information that confirms our own beliefs. This is all taking place in our subconscious. Professor of psychology at the University of Pennsylvania, Dr. Seth Gillihan stated, "Negative core beliefs can lie dormant when we're feeling well and emerge when we're gripped by strong emotions."[119]

For example, God tells me that I'm awesome and wonderfully put together (Psalm 139:14), but some kids at school have been calling me "ugly" since fourth grade, therefore, telling me I'm awesome and beautiful will make me feel an *uncomfortable internal inconsistency*.

To rid ourselves of the cognitive dissonance, our tendency is to take our belief and find evidence to support it. Using this example, to support my belief that I'm ugly all I have to do is look at some women's magazines. Then I'm 100% convinced that the models are prettier than me. This automatically reinforces my belief that I'm ugly. Then those uncomfortable feelings disappear because in my mind my false belief is confirmed, not God's truth (and I'll continue to self-sabotage).

"I'm ugly and always will be ugly" is difficult to turn around because not only are my beliefs being challenged, but so is my self-esteem and image. Think back to when you did the "The Power of 'I Am'" exercise (page 151). Were you comfortable telling yourself you were beautiful, valuable, awesome, beloved, brand new, etc.?

Feelings are not facts. Our emotions don't always accurately reflect reality and truth. This is why we need help and supernatural intervention, which we receive from God's Word, the Bible.

Hebrews 4:12 reads,

For the word of God is alive and powerful. It is sharper than the sharpest two-edged sword, cutting between soul and spirit, between joint and marrow. It exposes our innermost thoughts and desires.

This verse is telling us that when we read and ingest the Bible, the words penetrate deep within us and expose our hearts and motivations. The words in the Bible are not merely stored in your brain as data in some file. They are words that enter into your mind and heart with the power to transform your perceptions, emotions, decisions, principles, relationships, and your will. These words find their way into the secret places of your heart, giving wisdom, bringing courage and healing, whispering hope amidst the despair and sadness, and breaking each chain of bondage.

Even if we don't completely understand something in the Bible, we trust and follow God. God says to you: *"Call to me and I will answer you and tell you great and unsearchable things you do not know"* (Jeremiah 33:3). What an incredible promise!

Take the time each day to spend time with God in prayer (conversation) and experience the Bible and His *powerful living* Word. He will expose your predominant false beliefs and enable you to replace them with truth.

† Give a personal example of how your mind battles cognitive dissonance.

Part 1: Five Powerful Steps to Mind Freedom

We have power over what we believe and what we believe holds power over us—the power to thrive or be defeated. –Timothy Jennings, MD

What many of us fail to see is the abuser targeted and invaded our minds with lies, accusations and deceit. They have cunningly gotten us to believe our experiences are a result of our own inadequacies.

Remember: *I am the one who decides if another person's statement about me has power over me or not. Me only.*

Now is the time we take our minds back and embrace the cognitive dissonance. Did you know that two thoughts or emotions cannot occupy the same space? One always displaces the other. Have you noticed you can't worship God and be mad at the same time? It makes sense then we have to preload our minds with worship and good stuff.

The greatest power God gives us is the power to change our minds. *Thinking patterns and beliefs, and consequently lifestyle patterns, will only change with new input.* God wants to load a brand-new software program into your mind, one that He's designed specifically for you.

Doing these steps actually alters the brain's neuron and nerve cells, changing the way our brain works.[120] Commit to one, maybe two, steps per day. That's exciting!

Turn each step into a prayer request. Make it a conversation with Jesus. He must be at the center of this. Make each step a conversation with Him. As your Counselor, He is in this with you and will help you see on paper what's whirling around in your mind and soul—your reality.

> **Start: What is an emotion you're experiencing most profoundly that you want to deal with?**

If you're not sure, then think of a recent situation that seems to consume your mind, then name the strong emotion it evokes in you. "This situation makes me feel … anxious; ashamed; afraid; ticked-off; tormented; lonely; *however you are feeling."*

> **Step 1: What thought or belief comes to mind when I focus on how I'm feeling?**

Examples:
- *I feel furious* (burdensome feeling): Bob has always been so inconsiderate and still is (false belief).
- *I feel anxious:* "I'm a failure; not good enough; hopeless."

- *I feel ashamed:* "I'm bad. I didn't stop the abuse."
- *I feel frail and weak:* "I can't be that strong."
- *I feel scared:* "My boyfriend is going to leave me for someone else."
- *I feel lonely:* "No one understands what I'm going through."

Write out the thought just the way your mind is saying it. The goal is to recognize the thoughts that are tied to negative emotions.

Note: Some women struggle with the opposite of negative thoughts and beliefs; they're minds are filled with *superior, "holy," righteous and prideful thinking*. If you recognize this is you (often multiple people will point this out) then these are thoughts you need to work on.

Step 2: When I believe this thought, how do I feel and react?

Use these questions as a guide:

- Talk about any other *emotions* that arise when you believe that thought: the hurt, frustration, anxiety, rage, sadness, shame; whatever you're feeling.
- Is there a particular *image* that comes to your mind when you're [angry]? For example, a clenched fist.
- What *physical* sensations arise when you're [angry]? For example, blood pressure rises, experience insomnia, hands start to shake.
- How do you *act out* [the anger]? What coping or defense mechanisms do you tend to use?
- How do you *treat and talk to yourself* when you're [angry]?
- How do you *treat and talk to others* when you believe this thought?

Step 3: How might I—and my life—be different without this thought?

This is also a good time to ask God, "Do I need to forgive anyone?"

Most often this thought has become our identity and can be difficult to visualize who we'd be without it. By adding the power of our imagination, called "visualization" to a negative thought, we can move forward by rewriting an old mind script. One example: Visualize yourself stepping forward, towards Jesus, and stepping out of your fears, doubts, insecurities and woundedness.

In this step, take the time to visualize your future without this thought—visualize yourself living out the truth. Consider physiologically, emotionally and spiritually how you might feel. Relinquish the negative thought you have of yourself.

> **Step 4: Question and investigate the truth of the thought.**

We don't realize we have such strong negative core beliefs, until it's time to examine them. Instead of automatically finding evidence to support our negative core belief. We must put our core belief against the truth, which is the process of coming to an authentic conclusion.

This is what the disciple Thomas did when he said, *"Unless I see the nail marks in his hands and put my finger where the nails were, and put my hand into his side, I will not believe it" (John 20:25)*. It was also the reaction of Peter and John when Mary Magdalene told them Jesus's tomb was empty. They ran as fast as they could to the tomb to see firsthand if the report was true (despite the fact Jesus told them all He'd rise and come back).

We want to answer, to the best of our abilities, this question: *Can I be absolutely certain my belief is true? What kind of proof do I have this is absolutely true?* We ask God: *Does Your truth support this belief?*

We take the time to inquire, look for proof, and dig deeper. This is called "disputing." Ask God, *Am I looking at this all wrong? What are the facts?* We want to work with reality instead of false perceptions.

- Evidence supporting it is:
- Evidence contradicting it is:
- How accurate is my thought?
- Inaccurate: An alternative thought is:

If your belief is based on another person's remark, ask yourself and God: *"Based on this person's character and flaws, can he/she really be believed?"*

What if the negative belief is true? Stated belief: "My father has never loved me." In your investigation, you find out that your father intentionally distanced himself from you because you reminded him of his "awful and noxious" ex-wife, your mother. Unfortunately, this is true. Instead of believing all the reasons why your father shouldn't love you, seek reality. *Do not take his "stuff" on yourself.*

- Give yourself credit for having the courage to seek the truth. No matter the outcome, you are brave, open and on the right path.
- You now have an explanation as to why you think a certain way and do the things you do. You can continue to move forward.
- Ask yourself: "Ok. My dad never loved me. What's the worst that can happen?"
- Reflect on Dr. Lisa Najavits's comment, "The most painful truth is better in the long run than the most positive lie."[121]

Another thing we can do is ask ourselves (and Jesus), "What is another way to interpret this event—one that can generate more positive feelings about myself and those involved?"

Step 5: Create a new belief; a new truthful thinking track.

Thinking patterns and beliefs, and sleeping patterns, will not change without new input. Once we dispel the toxic thought and distance ourselves from it, then we have to replace it with something.

There's a saying in neuroscience: *Neurons that fire together wire together.* This means the more you run a neurocircuit in your brain, the stronger that circuit becomes. The more you practice something, the stronger those circuits get.

The Bible gives us precise instructions in Philippians 4:8 regarding restructuring our thoughts, which ultimately will reshape and transform our lives.

Whatever is true, whatever is noble, honorable, whatever is right, whatever is pure, whatever is lovely, whatever is admirable—if anything is excellent or praiseworthy—think about such things (Philippians 4:8).

The Message puts it this way:
I'd say you'll do best by filling your minds and meditating on things true, noble, reputable, authentic, compelling, gracious—the best, not the worst; the beautiful, not the ugly; things to praise, not things to curse.

These qualities are what I call "soul food" for the mind. *Whatever we focus upon increases,* which is why the phrase "think about such things" is critical. Notice the first quality mentioned to think on is truth. The challenge we have as Christians is to lay down a new set of default pathways that lead us naturally to think on that which is good, right, pure, and lovely.

Prayer and scripture are positive and productive, and can close down some negative thought files and create new positive files. I call this *deliberate rumination*—we continually focus on positive outcomes and changing our perspectives about ourselves, others and the world; we avoid seeing crises as insurmountable; we accept that loss and change are part of life, and focus on God and His plan.

Try these other exercises:

1—Turn a Harsh Thought into a Compassionate Thought

Example 1—Using the previous example, "My father never loved me," turns into "My father didn't love me—not because of who I am or what I did—but because he hated my mother so much. His lack of love has nothing to do with me. He needs to see a therapist and work out his issues with Mom. I have a heavenly Father who loves me so much. He wants to be part of my everyday life. He will never ever leave me."

Example 2—You believe, "I'm such a loser!" *If your best friend made the same statement, how would you answer her or him?* In other words, would you say you speak to yourself in the same way you do someone you respect and/or love, like your best friend or your child? Would you agree and tell her, "You're right! You're a huge failure"? No. You'd probably answer compassionately. Be your own best friend or child!

2—Redirect and Turn the Thought Around

Use the past tense when talking about your problem, and future tense when talking about how your life will be positively different. For example,

- Change *if* into *when:* "If I get out of this depression" becomes "When I get out of this depression."
- Change *can't* into *not yet:* "I can't stop drinking" becomes "I haven't stopped drinking yet."
- "I can't cope," becomes "I can do this through God's power."

Example: Maybe you've got a defective "man-picker," repeatedly choosing the wrong types of guys. For example, you can think, "I'll continue to choose guys who can't commit," or ask "How committed am I really? Have I healed adequately to be able to give and receive love?"

Consider this: We dislike, even hate, in others what we often dislike or hate in ourselves. It is easy to see the wrongs in others that we are equally guilty of (Matthew 7:5; Romans 2:1). Consider that a strong judgment about someone else, may be a cover up story we don't want to tell about ourselves.

Think of a couple of people you dislike or who irritate you. Might you have the same feelings buried deep in your unconscious about yourself? For example, "He should love me," turns around to "I should love myself." Or, "I can't live with this person any longer," turns around to "I can't live with myself any longer … and I need to gain some personal insight and healing."

3—Change a Belief about a Situation

We ask, *"Is the situation changeable?"* Not all are: 69% of circumstances involve unresolvable problems.[122] For example, Betsy's been trying to "fix" her sister's gambling addiction. She had to admit, "Darlene is never going to change without God's supernatural intervention. I can't fix her but I can pray for her." *We can change how we react to an unchangeable situation.* We reframe and change the *changeable;* what we have some control over. We let go of the *unchangeables* and turn them into prayers. For example,

Unchangeable (Prayer Request)	Makes Me Feel (Hopeless)	Changeable	Makes Me Feel (Hopeful)
Dad's controlling ways.	*I don't have a voice or a choice.*	I can set boundaries, speak up, follow God's lead and not dad's lead.	*Empowered.*
Ex-husband says I'll always be an addict and a failure.	*Like a loser.*	I can get clean; choose my destiny: go back to school, get training, find new friends, etc.	*Confident; worthy.*
5-year prison sentence.	*My life is over; I feel shamed, sometimes suicidal.*	I look at the sentence as an opportunity to grow, get clean, and take advantage of free programs.	*Like a conqueror; strong.*

Conclusion: Oswald Chambers wrote, "If a saint lets his or her mind alone, it will soon become a garbage patch for Satan's scarecrows." That's a word picture! Satan *will* deceive the mind that chooses not to think on truth. When we *know God,* then we can adequately program these qualities into our lives.

Personal Application: "I'm a failure."

What you believe is what you become ultimately. Too many women believe they are failures, and have similar beliefs of unworthiness. I want women to uncover the evidence they are not a failure through this example.

1—Write down your judgement statement about yourself—your thinking error. For example, *"I am a failure at everything I do."*

2—When I believe this thought, how do I react (the impact)? What do I do when I feel this feeling? How do I behave? *"Feeling like a failure makes me feel like if I do anything it will be wrong. I feel depressed, like I'm the only one who struggles with this. This is my core belief."*

3—How might I, and my life, be different without this thought? *"Without this thought I'd be a more peaceful and confident person. I'd feel free, like a huge weight has been lifted off my back. I'd be healthier too."* Picture who you'd be without this negative thought. *I see myself a successful missionary for God and a conqueror.*

4—Question and investigate the truth of the thought. *Can I be absolutely certain that it's true—that I'm a failure?* Naturally your statement appears true because it is based on a lifetime of uninvestigated unconscious beliefs. Your parents may have said so, therefore, you say so. But *can you be absolutely certain it's true that you're a failure? Or did you draw a wrong conclusion about yourself based on your parent's opinion, and not truthful reality?*

Look for the proof and inquire deeper. *Is there truth to support this belief? Did God's Word say I'm a failure?* Answer: No! Scripture proves that if I have God's nature in me, then I'm not a failure; not inferior, but a person of great value! God said that:

- I'm fearfully ("awesome") and brilliantly made (Psalm 139:14).
- I've been created for a specific purpose (Psalm 139:13-16); there's a special, divine blueprint for my life (Jeremiah 29:11).

- I'm a conqueror (Romans 8:37).
- God will complete through me what He's called me to do (Philippians 1:6).
- I have a spirit of power, love, and sound mind (2 Timothy 1:7).
- I can be conformed to the image of Christ—created to be a difference-maker in this world (Romans 8:29).
- "With Christ as my partner, there is no such thing as failure, only results" (Toni Sorenson).

To prove you're not a failure, focus your attention to some past successes you've had; and work with God to discover your unique blueprint. Write it all down. Look at everything you wrote. Then ask yourself if it's true that you're a failure; that you'll never amount to anything. The answer is NO! The evidence is clear and reveals your real worth.

5—Create a new belief; a new thinking track. Ask: *Can this thought be turned around? Can this situation be changed?* Yes. "I have special gifts and talents! I'm not a failure. There's something I can do that no one else can do! I've been chosen and appointed to bear good things (John 15:16)."

Part 2: Steps to Changing Painful Memories

> I was abused, raped, used drugs, and drank alcohol, all between the ages of 11 and 16. Getting a DUI scared me coz I almost killed someone. Right then I quit the drinking and drugs. But my past is still defining me. I find that old toxic thoughts and memories pop up out of nowhere. I get anxious and stomach aches. What's going on? –Kesha

Sigmund Freud once said, "I think this man is suffering from memories." Why are we triggered to think about, or dream about, our best friend from 1st grade who we haven't seen or heard from since grade school? The question I'd always ask is, "Why after decades does this person make another appearance in my dream world?" It's not like I thought about the person that day. My experience happened so long ago. Why are the memories still so strong when they're no longer relevant?

I'm not a neuroscientist but I do know: *Our brains don't forget.* The brain is like a computer that receives and retains data from the outside world. It compiles and maintains a record of *every* event. Scientists believe because women have a fairly larger *hippocampus*, they have better memories of the details of both pleasant and unpleasant emotional experiences[123]—which may be a blessing or a curse. My husband is astounded that I still remember—in detail—what he wore on our first date over 30 years ago.

Consider this: We are the most vulnerable when we are asleep. It is no surprise that feelings of abandonment, rejection, shame, etc. come up when we sleep. Past pains show up in our sleep—when we are at our most vulnerable. The solution is to take the dream to the light of day with safe people.

"Cannot be Deleted"

When you became a Christian, God deleted the file marked "sins," but there is no delete key for the files in your memory bank. Since your natural life is not obliterated, everything stored in your mind is still in there, written on your brain's hard drive.

Every experience and every trauma you've experienced has created an image, or memory, which is stored in your brain's visual center. Those images, and all the sensory data from those experiences, can arise anytime because the emotions about the event are still alive; they haven't been adequately processed.

For example, if as a young child you experienced a depressed, absent, or alcoholic parent whose moods couldn't be trusted awaiting you when you got home from school each day, then as an adult you might experience dread each day on your way home from work, and not understand that your sense of anxiety is connected to that experience.

Do you have a Facebook account? If you do then you're familiar with the "Memories" feature. If the memory post that pops up for that day is a pleasant one, it's not a big deal. But if the memory post is of your vacation with your ex, it can be the trigger to all sorts of unpleasant side effects—and nightmares. We can get flooded and blindsided with emotional and physical responses and symptoms.

The reason it's often difficult to forget when someone has hurt us is because the experience registers in the part of the brain designed not to reason, but to react.[124] The brain reminds us—physically and mentally—that this person caused pain, so it warns us to stay away. For the abused, the brain is super busy looking for confirmation that the world is a scary and dangerous place, and so are the people in it. These memories can lead to anxiety and other health issues.

Think of your memory bank as containing millions of recorded video-clips; a blueprint of your life. Every day of our lives, we make deposits in our memory banks. They affect us, our dream world, and write the scripts of self-talk. Ignoring them will not make them go away because each time one of those images arise, the neurological pathway strengthens, making it stronger.[125]

When we're drawn back repeatedly to the past without taking steps to heal, recovering from anxious and trauma memories can be difficult, if not impossible. Yet, God *"is able to do immeasurably more than all we ask or imagine, according to his power that is at work within us"* (Ephesians 3:20).

With God the word *impossible* turns into ***In-hiM-Possible.***

† Explain how you relate.

Revised Memories

Marlie recalled in 7th grade being grounded in her bedroom all day, on a Saturday, after mouthing off to her mom. She remembers spending endless hours in her room alone, bored and sorrowful. That's her memory. Then her sister tells her that they both got grounded, and their dad made them read the Book of John. Marlie didn't remember that piece of information, but she added it to this memory, thereby changing it.

Captured memories actually get revised all our lives. Our brain rewrites those memories over time based on new information and experiences. Each time we remember a trauma experience, that memory becomes susceptible to changes in how we remember what happened. We continually update, revise and rewrite some details based on new input and information, and erase other details. This is why it's important to be inputting truth rather than lies and false perceptions.

Interestingly, a memory is always attached to the same feelings we felt when the trauma experience first occurred, at whatever age we were. This is why 35-year-old Janet reexperiences her 5-year-old feeling of fear and helplessness when she thinks about or sees her grandpa, who molested her each time he bathed her.

Our brain constructs a world that no one can see, touch or hear. We store memories in two ways:

1. *Explicit memory:* Is a recollection of specific detailed events.
2. *Implicit memory:* Is the emotional sense of how the event made us feel; our gut responses.

Many of us who've had a trauma experience carry forward *implicit memories* of that experience even if we don't remember exactly what happened (*no explicit memory*). These emotional memories have a draw on us all our lives, often unconsciously. This is why it's important to work through toxic memories.

Reframing a Memory

Although we can't undo or erase a memory, we can weaken its impact significantly.[126] We can reshape and change them by building new truth-based memories. (Often professional counseling is required.) Let me explain.

Do you know why it feels so good to express pain to God and/or another person who empathizes with us? This is because it can buffer the effects of stress. Putting feelings into words diminishes the response in the *amygdala* (the part of the brain that handles fear, panic, and other strong emotions). I know I tend to feel calmer, better, and less fearful when I express how I truly feel.

Have you noticed "positive affirmations" and "positive psychology" are very popular today? Ever wonder why?

Neuropsychologists state that when two things are held in the mind at the same time, they start to connect with each other. That's why talking about hard things with someone who's supportive can be so healing: *The painful feelings and memories get infused with the comfort, encouragement and closeness you experience with the other person.* Therefore, positive experiences and declarations can be used to soothe, balance, and even replace negative ones.

Wendell Berry said, "We may strive, with good reason, to escape our past, or to escape what's bad in it, but we will escape it only by adding something better to it." This is why recovery groups are called recovery groups.

Memory Associations

If other things are in your mind at the same time that you call up a particular memory—and if they're strongly pleasant or unpleasant—the brain automatically puts them together—like two puzzle pieces. When this memory leaves the conscious, it is stored along with those other associations. The next time the memory is activated, *it will tend to bring those associations with it.*

We've all experienced eating something that we enjoy, but then we got sick (for whatever reason) and found we couldn't eat that food again. The good food memory turned into a bad food memory.

Another example: I asked my friend what she thought of the new pastor. I hadn't met him yet, but felt his sermons were strong and I liked his personality from the pulpit—*my memory of him*. She began spilling out a negative encounter she had with him. Immediately my impression of him changed—*I revised my memory*. The incidence didn't directly affect me, yet every time I saw him my mind would think he wasn't such a great pastor after all.

If we repeatedly bring to our minds, negative feelings and thoughts while a memory is active, then that memory will be saved and focused in a negative direction. Contrarily, each time you add positive information and feelings into negative and painful states of mind, *over time*, the accumulation of positive material will literally change your brain. This is because your incredible brain rewires itself by focusing attention on a new experience and encoding that image into its neural circuitry.

For example, by adding a memory of comfort, this may be enough to soothe us in a frightening situation. Pairing a memory of feeling connected to a safe and trustworthy person, for example, with an old memory of being abandoned, can enable us to thrive in future challenges.

Jon Kabat-Zinn wrote, "You can't stop the waves, but you can learn to surf." Since memories are being rewritten over and over again, we can learn how to rewrite them to empower us to move toward greater peace.[127]

Post-traumatic growth occurs when we work to change toxic memories by bringing in new, positive relevant information. When we redirect our thoughts onto things that are *true, good lovely, admirable, excellent or praiseworthy (Philippians 4:8)*, we will feel and perform much better. The result: *soul transforming peace*. ... Pairing a memory of feeling connected to a safe and trustworthy person, for example, with an old memory of being abandoned, can enable us to thrive in future challenges.

† What came up from your memory bank as you've digested this section of material?

Changing and Updating a Memory

When a bothersome memory surfaces, what we want to do is *update the memory*. We have two possible choices:

Choice #1: Update the memory by adding something **negative** (Unconscious Driven).

- *Mind develops an action plan to deal with a negative experience:* Ruminates on the experience →
- Adds a negative thought or image to the memory (Example: *This bad thing happened because I'm so stupid.*) →
- *Thinks:* "I need these bad feelings to go away. I know getting high will do this." →
- *Action:* Gets high and temporarily forgets. →
- Feels guilt and shame for drinking. →
- Creates new negative image. →
- Attaches to the old memory →
- Compounds past negative memory. →
- *Result:* Increased toxic thinking and destructive acting out.

Choice #2: Update the memory by adding something **positive** (Conscious Driven).

- *Mind develops an action plan:* Chooses *not* to ruminate on the negative experience →
- *Thinks:* "I need to be with someone who can console and listen to me," or "I need more information." →
- *Action:* Calls a friend or pastor; and/or gathers truthful and helpful information; and/or recalls a positive image. →
- Creates new positive image. →
- Attaches to old image/memory. →
- Minimizes toxic body/mind effects; changes present-day images.
- *Result:* The ability to "look back" at a disturbing memory from an empowered position.

Important: Unless we choose to work to alter our patterns of coping, we will always go to our unconscious default reactions.

Let me be clear: Updating our memories in no way takes away from the truth that a harmful event occurred, and that pain, sorrow and outrage may be significant components. And it certainly doesn't dismiss that a person who causes harm must be accountable for the offense.

Your Turn!
Recall a present-day situation where an intrusive memory or reaction from your past is disabling you from living in the present. Think of 2 to 3 pieces of positive information you can use to reframe and soften your reaction to the situation.

Example: Felicia's PTG Work
Adding new truthful, positive images to a sad, angry, tormenting or shameful memory can propel us out of that state and change the memory. Felicia needed to mourn losing her virginity. Let's follow her memory reframing process:

- I'm so sad I lost my virginity. I find myself ruminating on the rape, and my anger, and the unfairness at the loss of my innocence. → *Reframe to a truth-filled mindset* →

- I'm mourning the loss of not being able to experience a real "first time," and a feeling of closeness to my mate, as well as the experience of the awkwardness, the surprise, and excitement. → *Add a truthful, positive image to the memory* →

- I've learned that given my age and the circumstances, I was incapable of consenting. My step-dad committed a crime, yet he's made me feel imprisoned. I didn't give him permission to have sex me. My virginity was taken from me and that wasn't my fault. I was the victim. It's okay to feel sad and broken.
→ *Adds a truthful, positive image* →

- I also learned some people don't see a torn hymen as lost virginity. They believe it isn't a physical state but a spiritual, emotional, relational state; a state when the person gives consent and chooses to be with another person. Rape is not sex. It's an act of violence. They're not the same. I can experience the excitement and awkwardness of a "first time!" → *Adds another true positive image* →

- Since that awful day there have been many things I've done that were right, like breaking the secret! *The truth shall set you free! (John 8:32)*

Change Your Memory—Change Your Reality

You may also choose to use the 5-step formula to change a memory.

- *Step 1*—State your memory.
- *Step 2*—When I recall this memory, how do I feel and react?
- *Step 3*—How would my life change if I could change this memory?

Example: Jamie has many strong memories of her ex-husband controlling and emotionally abusing her. Jamie used "visualization" to prepare for a meeting with him. She expressed,

> In the past, when I had to meet with my ex, I'd become a wreck. All the old memories of his abuse came flooding out. So, I imagined myself strong; a powerful successful business woman. I saw myself walking into that meeting with my head high, shoulders back, and projecting tremendous confidence! Everything about me communicated I was strong, in control, and stable. I could feel my arms and legs and shoulder muscles; they were solid. I saw myself interacting with him competently—in complete control!

This new experience of empowerment, added to the old experience of being victimized, updated Jamie's memory of feeling overwhelmed and helpless in the face of her ex-husband with a new empowered image.

- *Step 4*—Question and investigate the memory.

- *Step 5*—Create a new memory by adding something "good" to it. We add a new positive experience; a new memory of comfort.

While we don't have the power to directly change our thoughts and emotions, we have the ability to change the image with which our emotions are associated. How? By *carefully choosing new experiences* that will help create new neural structures and rewire old brain pathways effectively and safely—thereby creating positive memories.

13

THINGS I WISH I'D KNOWN ABOUT LOVE

Have you ever made a "love-list" to help you find your ideal romantic partner? Brianna said, "I wrote up 55 characteristics and it had everything from dark denim jeans, to straight teeth, to 5'11" to 6'3" … all this detail."

Who doesn't long for a lasting, deep, passionate Cinderella kind of relationship? But, you've probably figured out there is no such thing as a gooey Hallmark Channel fairy tale ending.

Our vulnerability to the myth of Mr. Right comes from our glorification of romantic love. We receive messages all our life about what love is. Most of those messages are based on feelings and are lies because our culture has bred this Hollywood shallow and selfish view of love into us through the media and advertising.

The problem is many of us think that getting married will fill our soul hole and solve all our problems. I did. My only desire for going to college was to get a MRS. Degree (which I didn't receive). Many victims of abuse have an intense quest for affection. We long to be loved completely by someone who will never let us down. But we soon discover that this human being—no matter how well-intentioned—isn't capable of loving us perfectly. We might find someone, our prince, who makes us feel all tingly inside … for a short time. But this isn't real love. This view has contaminated the biblical meaning of love and sets us up to be vulnerable.

 According to professionals, the search for the perfect person to fix and complete us is truthfully delusional. Do you agree or disagree?

Fatal Attractions and Codependency

These past months have been the happiest times in my adult life. For the first time, I've forgotten my chaotic home. Everything, except Jeremy, faded into a blurry, silent background. As long as I have him, I know there will be no more pain. –Rennie

I always wondered why my love relationships ended up in what felt like a bloody battle. The answer: *An intense need for attention and reassurance*—which is why we give our hearts away so easily. We're running such a deficit in our love tanks that when we find what we think is real love, we give our hearts completely away. This is bondage, not freedom.

This lover will make my pain go away! When a dependent person chooses someone else to fill their void; to fill their internal security and sense of wellness, they create "relationship dependency." Unconsciously she says, "I can't love myself so you've got to love me for me." Words like *clingy, needy, suffocating* and *controlling* describe the relationship. Her mantra is, "Whatever you want. You decide for me." This is what we call a "need-love" mentality. When the person says, "I love you," she is really saying, "I need you. I want you to take something of yourself and fill the emptiness inside me with it."

My family had what I call "fuzzy" boundaries. My dad intruded into our lives, showing that he didn't honor us as individuals. He believed everything belonged to him which gave him the right to order us around. Unfortunately, people like me who come from these types of families struggle with independence and self-assurance; they feel more comfortable in dependent relationships that don't allow for much individuality.

Psychologist David Stoop wrote, "Because children from these families are not clear about boundaries, as they grow up they expose themselves to added hurt or exploitation in their attempts to build relationships."[128]

Most of us are what we call "relationally dependent" or "codependent." Somewhere we've learned that "alone" is not safe and we're not enough. We have a shattered self-image and low self-esteem, and then find ourselves connecting with others out of an unhealthy need to be loved, accepted, and/or to feel competent. Our built-in radars lead us to other half available persons in an attempt to make a whole person. We give control of our identities over to the other: "I need *you to define* who I am."

Relationship dependency (a.k.a. *Dependent Personality*) occurs when a person enmeshes an unhealthy self-identity with an equally unhealthy need for connection. It may be to a lover, spouse, friend, parent, or child. The person becomes dependent on the relationship to function in life. She will put up with the terrible because one, the alternative—being alone—is scarier and unthinkable, and two, to reduce the anxiety—all the while avoiding her own feelings and needs in relationship.[129]

If you were a victim of childhood abuse, chances are great you are relationship dependent. Abused children, unable to develop a sense of security, become more dependent than other children on external sources of comfort. Unable to develop a secure sense of independence, the child desperately seeks someone she can depend on. A fragmented inner sense prevents the development of a reliable sense of interdependence.

An abuse survivor is typically haunted by the fear of abandonment and/or exploitation. In a quest to be rescued, she may seek out powerful authority figures whom seem to offer the promise of a special caretaking relationship. If she can idealize her partner, then she can keep at bay the fear of being oppressed or betrayed. Unfortunately, she develops a pattern of intense and unstable relationships.

Dependent relationships are very powerful, seductive, and hard to resist due to the loyalty bonds which have been constructed (recall Stockholm Syndrome). Relational dependency can have a very dysfunctional face to it called *Betrayal or Trauma Bonding*. This is when a relationship develops into irrational loyalty or attachment. The focus on the other person is usually obsessive; meaning you're constantly preoccupied with the person—while neglecting to care for or value yourself.

Scientists who studied trauma in rats made a startling discovery. Rats that received electric-shock treatment in little boxes returned to those boxes when they experienced stress from other sources. Even though they received electrical shocks upon entering the boxes, they still returned to them. It was a familiar way to return to their known stress. Similarly, the trauma-bonded person will run back into the house of exploitation and abuse, even though it is toxic and dangerous.[130]

The search often leads to partners with complementary pathology: they both lack insight into their mutual destructiveness. One or both persons feel they cannot live complete without the other, nor walk out on the person. *Isn't this the definition of true love?* Not when each person encourages the other's dependency out of fear of being left alone.

It's like Siamese twins. If they attempt to break their attachment it feels like they're losing a part of themselves. This results in *enabling one another* and *resistance to separating* which is why so many remain in an abusive relationship.

I would add that if we have been living in "survival mode," just trying to cope and make it through each day, we may find ourselves at the opposite end of the spectrum—depending too much on ourselves.

Codependency and independency are the flesh's pull away from God, which according to the Bible is called *idolatry*. Profound disappointment is the cost when we put our trust in those who are merely God's creations. As humans, we can't love perfectly. We can, however, let our heartache lead us to the One who does know how to love us perfectly.

† Answer these questions. If you answer yes, explain:
- Do you thrive on being needed?

- Might you allocate too much time, attention, and value to another person, thereby, neglecting yourself and other people?
- Are you terrified of being alone?

Loving a High-conflict Personality

"Kimberly, there's a guy I want you to meet. His name is Bill and I think you guys will hit it off. He's charming and adorable. You'll love him!" This suave and good-looking guy, that my dear friend wanted me to hook up with, was not as he appeared. After spending over a year with him I'd describe him as toxic and dangerous; a parasite and a predator.

A *predator* seeks out victims, attempts to engage and build trust, then uses, oppresses, and exploits them. Bill was so calloused that he made me feel as though I were the one responsible for the pain he caused. Let me add, a high-conflict personality could also be a family member or friend or other person in our life.

Have you ever been in a relationship with this kind of person? Chances are, even if you were, you'd never know it. They're cunning charmers and master manipulators … and womanizers—to the point where we begin to accept the most extreme behavior as normal. These are extremely toxic people.

Some are "narcissists" and "sociopaths" (is an *antisocial personality disorder*); people who intentionally take advantage of and cause harm to others without any sense of remorse or responsibility. They lack a conscience, and their behaviors rapidly waver from one unhealthy extreme to another. They show no trace of empathy or genuine interest in bonding emotionally with a mate. Restraining orders are worthless. And their marriages are loveless and short-term.

As a Christian it is normal to want to redeem the unredeemable. Remember a personality disorder is exactly that—a disorder the person is saddled with. It can't be cured with a pill or logical conversation. We must decide to give them to God and let Him do His work.

Handling the Harasser

Don't engage in a war. Wars rarely end well because by definition someone will have to lose or die. –Gavin DeBecker

Terry called for weeks after I politely asked him not to. He left message after message, including threats. I found it hard to resist not responding and fighting him back. I thought if I could somehow make him stop, he would. The opposite happened. He only called me more. –Jackey

Victims of domestic abuse speak about a wonderfully romantic courtship ... then they'll describe the bomb that is dropped. Hence the term "love bomb." The combination of *seduction* and *fear* is a potent recipe used to distort the person's judgment. One psychologist said people are more sexually attractive to us when we associate them with danger. Reflect on that!

Gavin DeBecker has advised and protected political figures and celebrities from assassins, violent offenders and stalkers. He has the following advice on how to handle "harassers." He writes,

> There's an almost irresistible urge to do something dramatic in response to harassment and threats, but often, appearing to do *nothing* is the best plan. The only way you can have your desired outcome is to have *no contact*. As long as he gets a response from you, he is distracted from his own life.
>
> A strategy of watch and wait is usually the wisest step, but people frequently engage and enrage. The option of engaging a pursuer, once applied, simply means you can't go back to watch and wait. The minute you get into it with someone, you are into it. And if you get angry, that by itself is a victory for him.

This is a real test of patience and character for victims, but not responding often is the fastest way to end harassment. When a person requires something from us that is unattainable, it is time to stop negotiating because it's clear the person cannot be satisfied.

Believing that others will react as we would is the single most dangerous myth.

As long as you try to change the pursuer or satisfy him, it goes on. *Change what you can; stop trying to change what you cannot.*

I do want to say that "labels" (diagnoses) often imply that a person's identity is their psychological condition. I don't like the implied disrespect. For purposes of clarity and understanding, I've used these terms in this book as defined by the American Psychiatric Association's *Diagnostic and Statistical Manual of Mental Disorders.*

Let's not forget: Each person is made in the image of God and important to Him.

† Have you been in a relationship with this type of person? How did he/she make you feel? Perhaps at one time you were the "harasser"? How did that make you feel?

Being Single is Not a Curse

After everything I'd seen growing up, I knew I didn't want to get tangled in an abusive relationship or be with somebody who didn't want to really be with me. I made peace with the idea that I could live the rest of my life single. –Nicole

If you have a social media page then you know one of the profile statements requires stating your relationship status. A survey found 54% of the people lied about their relationship status on *Facebook*: 25% said they were in a relationship when they were actually single.[131]

Many of us have been indoctrinated to believe that if we're unmarried, we're a loser—a miserable misfit. We can all relate to the desire to find Mr. Right. Personally, the word *single* sounded to me like a disease. The fear of loneliness can be like a trap, luring the vulnerable into a predator's trap.

Some of us choose to be single for the wrong reason—we fear relationship pain. It's not the absence of people in our lives that releases us from pain. This is why we must choose to work on healing the pain-filled wounds and continue the growth process.

And there are those who have deep battle wounds think, "Men, I don't need them!" They believe building a permanent wall will protect them from future abuse. If you've been deeply hurt by a guy, let me say it is possible to enjoy the presence of a real, godly man. Meanwhile, enjoy the gift of singleness! Many women find a new strength and mission in being single ... and subsequently choose to stay single indefinitely.

Speaking about singleness, the apostle Paul said:

> *I'm not saying you must marry, but you certainly may if you wish. I wish everyone could get along without marrying, just as I do. But we are not all the same. God gives some the gift of a husband or wife, and others he gives the gift of being able to stay happily unmarried. So, I say to those who are widows—better to stay unmarried if you can, just as I am* (1 Corinthians 7:6-8).

Jesus said that when we're finally united with Him in eternity there will be no marriage to one another—only to Him (Mark 12:25). Also consider: Married people aren't the only heroes of the New and Old Testaments. What an example we have in the single lives of people like Jesus, Paul, Mary Magdalene and others.

Paul cherished his singleness because it put him utterly at the disposal of the Lord Jesus. No wife and children had to be taken into account when the mission for Christ was dangerous. He was not distracted by the needs of a spouse. No money had to be spent on clothing and educating little Paul or Paula. Living a holy life as a single person is a high calling, one that many people choose willingly.

Being Alone Is Okay
"Mr. Right" sometimes appears as "Mr. Wrong" but we blow it because we're seeking a delusional image. Please do not suffer another horrible relationship for fear of being alone. *A survivor must move into interdependence.* Remember—you are not alone; never: *"For the LORD your God goes with you; He'll never leave you nor forsake you"* (*Deuteronomy 31:6*).

The process begins with accepting reality. It is the essential factor of having a healthy relationship with ourselves. Henri Nouwen calls the transition the "conversion of loneliness into solitude."

Michaela said, "A lot of people, especially shrinks, assume happiness can only be found in a couple. But not all of us are made for coupling." Singleness can be a gift. Advantages of being single are: A greater focus on Christ; a larger area of influence on other people's lives; the ability to give away our free time and spiritual gifts. As a believer, none of us is really single; we're already in a relationship with Jesus.

† Explain how you now feel differently about singleness?

Relationship Restoration Plan

Love demands a great amount of respect for the other person as an individual, and it is based on autonomy not a blending of personalities. Love is not found by fitting one person into another's mold, and it is not a question of finding the perfect "match." It is a union with somebody outside oneself, under the condition of retaining the separateness and integrity of one's own self. –Erich Fromm, PhD

As a married woman, there have been *numerous* times in my relationship when I felt God made a mistake joining my husband and myself together. Now after 25-plus years of marriage I can certainly say that committed relationships provide us with the maximum opportunity for growth. When my husband is pushing all my buttons, he is making me grow by learning how to be patient and humble. ("Pushing buttons" isn't the same as being abusive but describes a relationship with normal marital conflict.)

Lastly, most marriage experts say a good marriage is built on *friendship* first in which *the power is shared*. And what we know is that "true" loving friends keep their friendships going for a lifetime because they don't indulge in fantasies of ownership.

A healthy relationship can be described as two good friends becoming better friends and growing. The strongest and most successful relationships, even the most passionate and romantic marriages, have this kind of true friendship as the foundation. Ask yourself, "If I were not hormonally attracted to this person, would he be someone I'd enjoy as a friend?" If the answer is no, there's little chance for that love to succeed.

Proverbs 18:24 states, *"A man of many companions may come to ruin, but there is a friend who sticks closer than a brother"* *(ESV)*. When the foundation of true friendship is absent, the relationship is shallow and susceptible to being marked by *victimization (suffering from a destructive or harmful action)*.

Good news: Because our brains are wired to change, we can be in a healthy non-dependent growing relationship. The opposite of codependence is "interdependent," which *doesn't* mean "I don't need anybody. I can make it on my own." It means to *depend on others in a healthy way*. For example, I depend on my husband to bring home a paycheck. He depends on me to grocery shop for the family.

We are responsible *to* each other, but not *for* each other. Scripture says to *"Bear one another's burdens" (Galatians 6:2)*. Then three verses later it says, *"For all must carry their own loads" (v. 5)*. The point: When we see another's need, we are to support them, not enable them. Two persons can become one without losing their identities.

Characteristics of Interdependent People

How do we grow a godly relationship? Not by asking God to change our partners, but by asking God to change our minds. God is the only One who can truly change our spouses, (and parents, family members, or friends). We're not to rescue, fix, enable, or attempt to take God's place. Our responsibility is to lovingly point them to Jesus, and then trust Him to do His work.

A healthy interdependent relationship has the following characteristics:

- God is #1 in the person's life. Marriage is God's gift to a man and woman, a gift that should be given back to Him.
- They are independent; can separate; share feelings; know where proper boundaries begin and end; and be flexible.
- They refuse to rescue or enable the behavior of their partners.
- They set limits on their partner's destructive acts or attitudes and allow them to experience the consequences.
- They don't try to solve the other person's problems; instead they encourage them, helping to make them stronger.
- They can compromise and reach a mutual agreement.
- They know their "true self" and don't have any expectations that another person can complete them. One person may be strong in some situations, and weak in others.
- They *respect* and *adore* one another. (In general, a man's desire is to be respected, and a woman desires to be adored.)
- They develop creative coping and conflict resolution skills.
- They make use of support people and systems.
- They *trust* and *accept* each other just the way they are.

A committed relationship is like a flowering bush. In its season, the blossoms fall off. But if the plant is well nourished and kept, the next season it will bloom again. We all have seasons when the blooms fall off. Our soul mate is a human being like we are. He too is going through continual growth. No one is ever finished or "complete."

When there is conflict, healthy partners try to work things out. Other times, the lesson to be learned is how to exit lovingly and gracefully. If a breakup occurs, separation is seen as a new chapter. The person can say, "I love you so much that I can release you to be where God needs you to be."

14

RECEIVING THE RIGHT KIND OF LOVE

He manipulated my gift of love in order to cause me pain! I mean, who does that? I need to know what real love is and how to avoid toxic people so this will never happen again. –Pennie

To love people is risky. The greater the love, the greater the risk. This is why God has given us *1 Corinthians 13,* which is His clearest picture of what an intimate love relationship is.

The Greeks had multiple definitions of the word "love." In the New Testament, the word "agape" is one translation of "love" which is the word used in this passage. Unlike our English word for love, *agape* doesn't refer to romantic or sexual love.

Agape love is an "unselfish, thoughtful, unconditional, sacrificial love which doesn't expect anything in return." It's the kind of love a mother has for her child. For many, it escapes human comprehension. It's the opposite of a dependent "need-love" mentality. God agape loves us, and agape love is how God created us to live and love others. It is a supernatural love—a love from God.

Have you read Francine Rivers's book *Redeeming Love?* It is a romance story about a prostitute named Angel and a godly farmer named Michael Hosea—based on the Old Testament book of Hosea. *Redeeming Love* is set during the Gold Rush of 1850, a time when greed flourished. Angel was sold into prostitution as a child. She has no interest in God or religion. She distrusts all men who see her only as an object to satisfy their lust.

Michael Hosea is a devout Christian. He is told by God to marry this soiled dove. He said, "She's the one," the woman he's meant to marry. When he discovers that Angel's a prostitute (can you imagine?), surprisingly, Michael is still determined to go through with

God's command to marry Angel. (This reminded me of Joseph who obeyed God and married the pregnant Mary, mother of Jesus.)

Michael paid the fee for Angel's time in hopes of convincing her to leave with him, but she rejects his offer. Discouraged, Michael questions God's command, but still moves on in obedience. He goes back and pays Angel's fee for three successive nights. He spends the entire time talking and reasoning with her.

Despite Michael's earnest efforts, Angel hangs on to her cold, sarcastic front ... but, like a true love story, she can't seem to get Michael out of her mind ... and also the hope of a life on the outside.

After being badly beaten, Angel decides to take Michael up on his offer of marriage. Michael nurses Angel back to health and she begins to hope again, but is soon overwhelmed by fear. So, she runs away from Michael and returns to her old life. Even though she loathes being seen as nothing but a whore, she knows she has no other skills with which to make a living.

Michael continues to pursue her. One day he finds her in a room with a client. Like a true hero, he grabs her and fights their way out of a smoky bar filled with drunken men who are all waiting for their turn with Angel.

Michael takes her to his cabin and finds himself relying on God to work through his anger at her unfaithfulness (not surprising). Angel finally begins developing feelings towards Michael, which she can't comprehend because she's never allowed herself to love any man. Despite her continued coldness and lack of heart, Michael loves her unconditionally. Eventually, Angel learns not only to love Michael, but to love God too.

Michael shows us the true meaning of agape love. *It is a decision, versus a feeling—similar to the forgiveness process.* The book of Hosea is a beautiful picture of God's unconditional love for His people, no matter what they do.

The Agape Love Chapter:
1 Corinthians 13:4-9

Love is patient, love is kind. It does not envy, it does not boast, It's not proud. It's not rude, It's not self-seeking, It's not easily angered, it keeps no record of wrongs. Love does not delight in evil but rejoices with the truth. It always protects, always trusts, always hopes, always perseveres (1 Corinthians 13:4-9).

The Message version reads: *"Love never gives up. Love cares more for others than for self. Love doesn't want what it doesn't have. Love doesn't strut, Doesn't have a swelled head, Doesn't force itself on others, Isn't always 'me first,' Doesn't fly off the handle, Doesn't keep score of the sins of others, Doesn't revel when others grovel, Takes pleasure in the flowering of truth, Puts up with anything, Trusts God always, Always looks for the best, Never looks back, But keeps going to the end. Love never dies."*

I would add: *"Love is not controlling; does not exert power over."* This passage is driven by the principle of love. This kind of love is bigger than our emotions. Notice it summarizes the *behaviors of love*. "Gooey" love feelings don't last nor sustain a love relationship; behaviors do. Love is defined by making loving behavioral choices. It means taking care of your partner's needs before your own, whether you feel like it or not.

No person can behave completely like this, unless imparted by Jesus. He is *the Source*. Yet, both people should desire and strive to meet these qualities. Practice makes perfect as they say!

I'm going to be bold and say that if the person you love expresses and lives out the *opposite* of each of these characteristics, such as extreme jealousy, possessiveness, anger, distrust, self-centeredness, is demeaning or depresses you, you're in dangerous territory. His focus should be on how he can serve you, instead of on you serving him.

Let me speak to "Love doesn't keep a record of wrongs." Some women say, "The Bible says *'love covers a multitude of sins; it covers all wrongs!'" (1 Peter 4:8)* In other words, "I love you so your bad behavior is okay. I'm going to expunge your records of wrongs." Love does cover a multitude of sins—but not all sins. Serious and repetitive sin is lethal to any relationship and should not be covered up. Then it becomes a "cover up."

In her book *The Emotionally Destructive Marriage,* Leslie Vernick wrote, "Maybe you think that God is more interested in preserving your marriage than the well-being of you and your children, but that's not true. God values marriage, but he's also concerned for your safety and sanity in the midst of a destructive/and or dangerous marriage."

Forgiveness doesn't mean we eliminate accountability and consequences or pacify a relationship just to keep the peace. This is called "pseudo peace." (1 John 3:6-10.) Proverbs 19:19 states, *"A hot-tempered man must pay the penalty; if you rescue him, you will have to do it again."* The best way we can love someone is to hold them accountable for their actions. In the psychology field they have a saying, "Past behavior is the best predictor of future behavior."

Lastly, "love never dies" means love never ends; it has staying power. It's when two people honor each other's values, standards, and purpose. Like God's love, our love—our actions—should benefit the other person, regardless of the cost or feelings. They don't just talk about it. They live it. They "do" love. Real love says, "I've seen the ugly parts of you and I don't think any less of you!"

If you are in a romantic relationship ask, "How does the man I love, and who claims to love me, measure up to God's definition of love? Does this person create harmony or chaos?" And more importantly, "Is this person connected to the Source of love?"

What you will receive from this person will be only as good as their connection to Jesus.

The *ABCDE's of agape love*:
- I **A**ccept you as you are.
- I **B**elieve you are valuable.
- I **C**are when you hurt.
- I **D**esire only what's best for you.
- I will **E**ndure through all things with you.

Biblical Submission = Equality

"Submission" is a four-letter word in our culture. We resist anything or anyone who limits our personal freedom. We equate submission with weakness, don't we? In God's culture submitting to His plan for us doesn't mean we're weak or imprisoned. It means we're free.

The Bible says, "*It is for freedom that Christ has set us free* [past tense]. *Stand firm, then,* [present tense] *and do not let yourselves be burdened again* [like in your past life] *by a yoke of slavery*" (*Galatians 5:1*).

God originally designed His created to be free—not to be enslaved by another person or by each other, but to love each other freely. Any violation of God's law of love damages our ability to love.

Where there is power and control in a relationship, or the perception of power and control, there is no love, only bondage. Love only exists where there is a spirit of freedom. Dr. William Glasser wrote, "It is hard, if not impossible, to love someone you want to control and change."[132] Freedom is necessary for love to develop. Freedom creates a safe and secure environment for a couple to love, trust, explore, and deepen their experience of each other. Each person is free from the other, and therefore, free to love the other.

Many women are accustomed to accommodating their partner's desires and freely give away power and choice in relationships. If what you've experienced in an intimate relationship doesn't line up with what God says love and submission is, then it's not love; it's most likely "oppression."

Abusive men have an uncanny ability to carry out their power and control tactics while at the same time pretending to be in love. The effect on the woman is that she takes whatever roles are assigned to her. She is denied equality.

According to Dr. Glasser, it's rarely the lack of love that destroys relationships; it's more that love cannot take root in a relationship in which one or both partners believe they have too little or no power.[133]

God said, "*It is not good for the man to be alone. I will make a helper suitable for him*" (*Genesis 2:18*). "Helper" is the opposite of "slave." The

Bible is clear that both male and female are created equal. Whatever is true about the image of God in a man is true about the image of God in a woman. Every woman was created by God equal to man. The female is made of the same spiritual stuff as the male.

Article I of the Universal Declaration of Human Rights states: *All human beings are born free and equal in dignity and rights. They are endowed with reason and conscience and should act towards one another in a spirit of brotherhood.*

✝ When have you been made to feel fully equal in a relationship?

Submission versus Oppression

Show proper respect to everyone. –Peter, speaking in 1 Peter 2:17

Let's look at the difference between *godly submission* and *unrighteous oppression*.

The word "submit" is one of the most difficult, disliked, and divisive words in the Bible. "Submit" means to *willingly* line up under another's authority. Submission is an act of a person's free will. This means I voluntarily yield and limit what I naturally desire to do in this relationship in order to benefit you. Submission *isn't* about following "orders." It isn't translated as, "Do what I say" or "Just do it!"

Ephesians 5:21 gives us a command: *"Submit to one another out of reverence for Christ."* Here the word submit means "accommodate to" or "give way to." Let's say that I'm the one with more power (for example, I make a lot of money); instead of using that power (money) to make my life easier, out of admiration and respect for Christ, I'll use my power (money) to serve and empower you. I'm willing to give up things I want in order to benefit you. On the other hand, if I'm the one with less power, submission means that instead of doing what I might do naturally, like fight you every step of the way, I choose to respect and honor your decisions.

Dr. Gregory Jantz wrote, "The power to demand obedience is a great responsibility. When we obey others, we submit to their will above our own. Therefore, this power should be used sparingly and only with the other person's best interests in mind."

On earth, Jesus submitted. He gave up His position and power in order to fulfill God's mission. Even today, He doesn't insist on having control or authority over us. He never says, "You'll submit to me! You must do it My way!" He gives us the choice if we want to follow Him or not.

Abusive and self-centered men do the opposite. They twist the gift of submission to manipulate and control the other person into doing what they want, thereby, creating an unjust power imbalance called "oppression" which is *the exercise of authority or power in a burdensome, cruel, or unjust manner; the feeling of being heavily weighed down, mentally or physically, by troubles, adverse conditions, anxiety, and the like.*[134]

Oppressive people demand others see and do things their way, bowing to their authoritarian ways. Their love is not self-sacrificing; it's self-gratifying. Think of oppression as *demanded submission.*

Any type of headship that results in violent, controlling, or fear-based power and control is *not* biblical. God designed love so there will be no fear; no loss of freedom, for *"perfect [agape] love casts out fear" (1 John 4:18).*

It's our misunderstanding of what submission is that causes us to back down or give in—even when we know deep down the action is wrong and doesn't please God. *"The LORD works righteousness and justice for all the oppressed" (Psalm 103:6).*

† What have you been taught or believed about "submission"?

Gender Equality

Women hold up half the sky. –a proverb

God is clear: Women are one of the world's most precious resources! Both Jesus and the early church elevated women.[135] He created man in His own image; both male and female. He gave both sexes the exact same responsibilities (Genesis 1:27-28). The Bible records God's intentionality to reestablish the position of women to that of equality with men.

God's Son, Jesus Christ, not only bridged the gap between God and man through His death on the cross; He removed all barriers including that of gender, race, and nationality. The way Jesus acted towards women was revolutionary and shocking. Relaxed and open with women, Jesus allowed them to touch and kiss Him, a rabbi. Accepting, sensitive, and affirming, He treated all women with the deepest respect. He's the kind of man God wants every woman to know. You can trust Jesus with your heart.

Ephesians 5:25 states, *"Husbands, love your wives, just as Christ loved the church and gave himself up for her,"* God is telling husbands to give up their position, power, and their own way in order to minister to and love their wives. The husband is to be a Christlike example to his family. He should be the leader in being compassionate, kind, forgiving, and all the other attributes Jesus lived out, especially love.

This passage says the husband is the head of the wife. Does this make him the boss and give him the role of unquestioned authority? No, it makes him the "head servant." We come to this conclusion because Jesus said He *"did not come to be served, but to serve"* (Matthew 20:28).

The word "head" in this passage means the husband is to put aside his own interests in order to care for his wife. *Headship is not dictatorship.* The word "love" in this passage means "to cherish; to nourish or rear up to maturity." It's not a statement of power and control. The husband is not to "use" his wife for his own pleasure, but rather show the kind of love which is mutually rewarding.

Paul had more to say to the Christian husbands than to the wives. He set a high standard for them to follow—to love their wives as much as Christ loves them and all His children (the Church). If he does, then he loves her sacrificially and *will not desire* to oppress her.

When a wife submits to Christ first, and lets Him be the Lord of her life, she should have no difficulty submitting to her husband because the husband and God act together. This doesn't mean she becomes his slave—for the husband is also to submit to Christ. If both are living under His lordship, there will be harmony.

When we take a marriage vow, we are agreeing to leave behind our life as two separate individuals and enter into a new union: something mystical and magical. It's the death of our independence. We leave behind our self-sufficiencies. Life together is as "one"—which is a picture of the gospel.

Regarding sexual abuse: Depending on the degree and kind of abuse you suffered, you may need time to work through sexual triggers. A truly good husband will give you as much time as you need. He will communicate and empathize, ensuring you feel comfortable no matter what. Instead of sex being used for manipulation, you'll find that normal, healthy partners have sex the way God designed it—to intimately and express agape love for one another (Genesis 2:24).

† Submitting to Christ first enables us to submit to others. We find joy in submitting to others when we know that it is to Jesus that we ultimately submit. Would you say you are fully submitted to Jesus? Or a work in progress (like me)? Explain.

Take Control with Boundaries

No study on restoration from abuse is complete until we speak about boundaries. Because someone with more power invaded our personal space and stepped over the line, we may be uncertain how to set limits today. As bad as it is for adults to cross that line, it's more traumatic for children. Their limits haven't been fully formed which leaves them confused.

When I read this response by a guy named Peter, I could have sworn he was writing about me. Perhaps you too can relate. Speaking of his girlfriend,

In the beginning, she was like a breath of fresh air. But as time went on, I could never figure out what she wanted. I would ask her what she wanted to do, or where she wanted to go, or how she felt about something, and she'd always defer to me. Even though that felt good in the beginning, over time, I felt something missing. I was also frustrated not knowing when things were okay and when they weren't. I need someone who knows what they are thinking and what they want.

Here's another scenario you may relate to: Deidre and Mike had been dating for almost a year. When her opinion was the same as his, things were fine. But, whenever Deidre expressed an opinion that didn't match Mike's, he'd become irate. Consequently, Deidre began to withhold her opinions which meant she could no longer be herself. She couldn't talk about certain subjects because Mike challenged and belittled her.

Over time, Deidre shifted what she wanted to what he wanted in order to please him and gain his approval. Eventually, with the help of friends, she identified the problem—Mike's behavior. Then Deidre stood her ground. When Mike discovered he could no longer control her, he broke up with her.

Deirdre learned: *We teach people how to treat us by our response to them.*

Drs. John Townsend and Henry Cloud wrote,

> Many people think of boundaries only as setting limits, saying no, or trying to stop something destructive from happening. But having good boundaries is more than stopping bad things from happening to you. It is also taking responsibility for the good things you want to happen. We need to own our "want"—be honest about what we want and own our desires; own our feelings—if we're sad, we need to say so, and not wait for the other person to figure it out.[136]

Boundaries are limits set to help protect us. The offending person needs to feel the weight of what they've done and own their behavior. Setting a boundary can be as simple as "That doesn't work for me." You don't need to justify nor feel bad or fearful or guilty. In fact, *rejoice in the guilty feelings!* How does that statement make you feel?

As strange as it may seem, a sign that you're becoming a boundaried person is often a sense of guilt, or a feeling that you've broken some important rule. This is normal when we begin telling ourselves the truth about *what is* and *what isn't* our responsibility. It is an important step in separating from high-conflict people and affirming our voice. An old Indian proverb goes, "People can only walk on your back if you're bent over."

† Finish this sentence: "When setting a boundary, I rejoice in my guilty feelings because …"

No is a Complete Sentence

The Bible contains admonitions for us to separate ourselves from fellow Christians who act in destructive ways (Matthew 18:15–17; 1 Corinthians 5:9–13). If we do this, we are not being unloving. Separating ourselves protects love because we are taking a stand against things that destroy love.

We really can't set limits on others; in that we cannot control them. What we can do is set limits on our own exposure to people who are behaving poorly; we can't change them or make them behave correctly.

Boundary-busters can only get their way when we accommodate them, usually because we want their approval so desperately. Jesus said, *"All you need to say is simply 'Yes' or 'No'; anything beyond this comes from the evil one"* (Matthew 5:37).

Any time you feel uncomfortable learn to say "No." Period. Say it calmly. You don't need to explain or justify your no. Because you're entitled to love and a good life, take a stand: either the abusive person treats you as you deserve or choose to walk away. You may say something like,

- No, I'm not going to join in this conversation. I'm opting out.
- Mom, your laughing at me hurts my feelings. While you do it, I'm choosing not to talk to you.
- No, I don't feel comfortable with that. No, I won't do that."

Raise an Issue in A Non-Blaming Way

Nothing is guaranteed to provoke a fight faster than being highly reactive and telling someone "You *always* do ...," "You're attacking me," or "You're acting like a hoodlum." The best way is to raise an issue in a non-blaming way is by focusing on yourself. Clarify and define yourself:

- I know this is a stressful time for you but I feel that you're attacking me.
- It's hard for me to hear you call me names. That's how I feel.
- I have a rule for those who live in this house which is ...
- I want you to tell me how you think we're doing in our relationship.

Saying *"I" and "me"* diffuses the possibility the other person will get defensive or will choose to leave the conversation. Use "I" statements: *"I feel," "I think," "I want," "I need," "I have."*

Focusing on our feelings instead of pointing the finger at someone else will almost always decrease defensiveness and opposition. If he/she doesn't respect your wishes, you may just have to completely opt-out and shut down the conversation.

Secondly, if we are dealing with someone with a personality disorder, according to experts, we should respond with empathy, attention, and respect. For example,

I can see you feel frustrated. [Empathy] *I want to hear from your point of view.* [Attention] *I respect you for your desire to solve this problem.* [Respect][137]

This person will likely have difficulty taking no for an answer, or believing any boundary applies to them. That's why we have to back up our limits with clear consequences.

Stopping the Dance

Your first responsibility is to yourself and loved ones. Don't let anyone tell you that you must stay in a relationship where you will be bullied, tormented, exploited, or victimized. God never says this.

- Don't ask yourself "Who's right?" Ask yourself, "Do I like being treated this way?"
- Don't debate what you know to be true. *Trust your gut!*
- Always tell yourself the truth—about yourself and the situation.
- Practice and role play opting out of arguments:
    o *I'm happy to continue talking, but without the name calling.*
    o *I think we have to agree to disagree.*
    o *I love talking with you, but not when you're putting me down.*

Define the Consequences

Boundaries without consequences are worthless. As a God of justice, He sets boundaries. Due to His people's cyclical pattern of disobedience, they lost the inheritance of the promised land. Through countless judges, prophets, and other leaders, God repeatedly warned His people to turn back to Him. But they abandoned Him, causing God to allow them to be taken captive.

Don't set a boundary unless you are willing to follow through with a consequence. Learning how to set boundaries is to learn how to set and stick with consequences—and be a united front, if two or more people are involved in setting them.

A boundary without a consequence isn't worth much. This only enables the person to take over your life. God sets consequences for certain behaviors. If you have children, you (should) understand this concept. Examples are:

- I feel your behavior is dangerous. If you can't stop, for the safety of myself and the kids, I'll leave until you get treatment.
- I cannot allow you to stay here if you continue to criticize me.
- I'm not a money tree. I can't give you more money if you quit another job without lining up another one.

† Why do you think your number-one boundary-buster keeps breaking your boundaries? How can you turn this situation around?

Choose Your Battles

I am sending you out like sheep among wolves. Therefore, be as shrewd as snakes and as innocent as doves. Be on your guard. –Jesus, speaking in *Matthew 10:16-17)*

Trust your instincts. Be discerning and selective in who and what you allow in your life. You deserve a relationship in which you feel safe and respected. Proverbs 4:23 states, *"Above all else, guard your heart, for it is the wellspring of life."* (Notice the emphasis *"above all else"* …)

When we *do not guard* our hearts, we're choosing to go to war. If you find yourself in a toxic relationship but are having trouble with setting what you know to be healthy boundaries, ask yourself: Do I feel anxious, not like my normal self; depressed or like I'm living in a chaotic emotional tornado? Professionals say: Always trust and go with your instincts and anxieties.

If you are in a relationship with a high-conflict person and you state your limits, often all they will hear is rejection. Experts say to stay calm and not escalate your emotions, communicate in a way that you'd like them to mirror, avoid threatening language, and be consistent.

Jesus said we will know a good tree by its fruit and a diseased tree by the fruit it bears (Matthew 7:17). When you believe you've picked the perfect mate and are ready to get married, I plead with you both to invest time in getting to know one another (at least one year) and do pre-marital counseling. According to Psychology Today, studies suggest that couples that choose to receive pre-marital counseling have lower divorce rates than those that do not. Most churches offer this and may even require it if you want to be married in the church.

15

OUR FINAL MOMENT

Forget the former things; do not dwell on the past. See, I am doing a new thing! Now it springs up ... —Isaiah 43:18-19

Childhood abuse, sexual assault, intimate partner violence, and rape are words that have been broadcasted on the news and social media outlets in the wake of the #MeToo movement. People all across America have shared their most vulnerable and tragic moments. The impact of women who have come forward to share their stories has changed the trajectory of the way our culture views sexual harassment. The "face" of a perpetrator is no longer "creepy" but the person on the morning news, or our kid's soccer coach, even the guy at church.

These women have incredible courage to share their stories. They carried immense weight of the trauma into the public eye. You too have shown immense courage in completing this study. This is quite an accomplishment. There's an excitement in heaven I believe.

Share in Paul's joy, *"I have fought the good fight, I have finished the race, I have kept the faith"* (2 Timothy 4:7). It's been rough, but your courage and faith in God got you through. No doubt, God has brought hope and healing into your life and demolished some big strongholds. Praise Him for that.

Before Mother Teresa died, she said, "I have worked for God all my life and I know I will soon be dancing in heaven. I wish I had danced more during my time on earth."

Go and dance in the Sonshine!

Appendix A

THE FEELING WHEEL

Identified or labeled feelings are manageable; unidentified emotions can feel overwhelming. Use this chart to identify exactly how you feel. Ask Jesus to help you clarify your feelings.

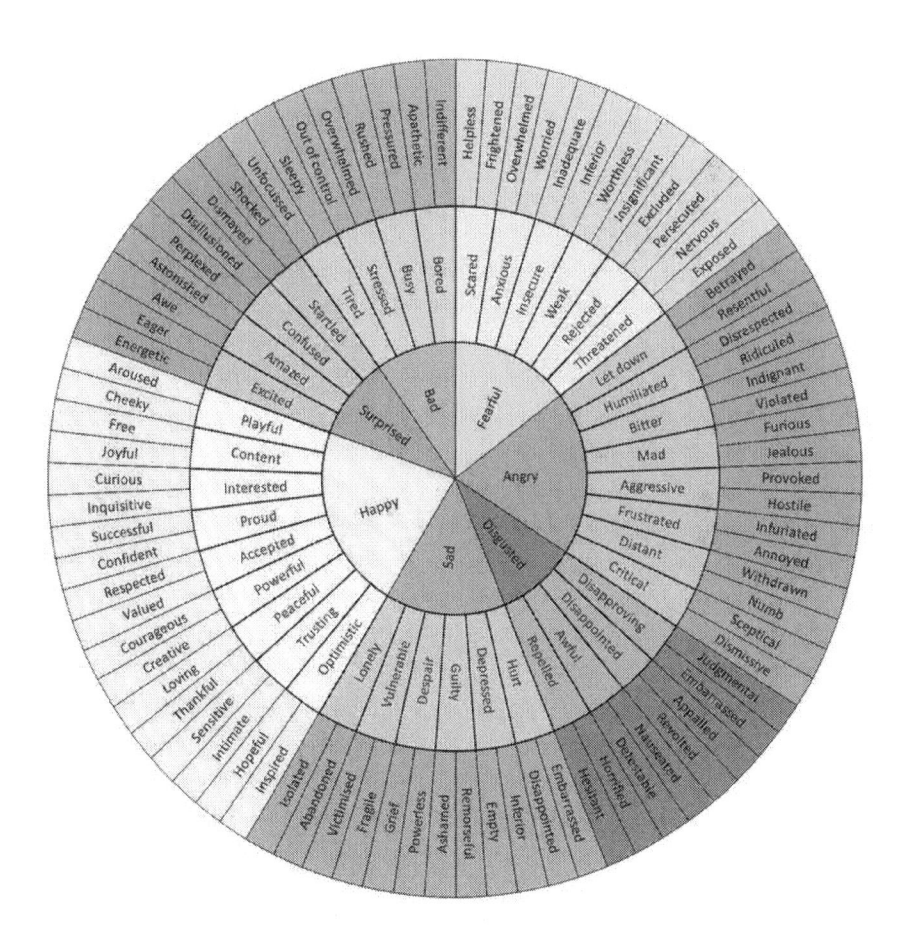

Appendix B

Deep Breathing

"Slow down. Take a breath. What's the hurry? Why wear yourself out?"
—Jeremiah, speaking in Jeremiah 2:25 (MSG)

The material and the exercises in this book are tough. It's important we care for ourselves as we go through each chapter. We can befriend any anxiety through practicing deep breathing exercises which can help anchor us in the present moment. Breathing exercises oxygenate the blood and the cells, supporting all life-giving biological pathways and move energy. It is a great way to de-stress and relax deeply and move any stuck feelings in the body or mind. It can reduce anxiety, bring you into the present moment through mindfulness, and help you remember how to respond to your specific stressors, and move any stuck feelings in the body or mind. It's a pretty incredible healing exercise.

Deep breathing (a.k.a. *abdominal breathing; belly breathing*) is when you breathe deeply; the air coming in through your nose fully fills your lungs, and the lower belly rises.

When people are stressed, they tend to breathe shallowly from their chests rather than their stomachs. Deep breathing from our stomach activates a different brain pathway which causes the brain and body to calm down. Once engaged in deep breathing, we feel it slow down our racing minds and calm us down.

The professionals agree that to overcome the unhealthy day-to-day stress response, we should practice this type of breathing daily, regardless if we're feeling stressed because it can prevent the stress response from overacting in the first place.

When starting out, put aside a few minutes, once or twice a day, to slow down your breath.

- Find a quiet, comfortable place to sit or lie down.
- First, take *a normal breath* and relax.
- Place one hand on your chest and the other on your stomach.
- Breathe normally. Focus on feeling your chest rise.
- Breathe in slowly through your nose, allowing your chest and lower belly to rise as you fill your lungs. Let your abdomen expand fully. Feel your hand rise.
- Now slowly *take 3 deep breaths*: 1—2—3. Breathe out slowly through your mouth (or your nose, if that feels more natural).
- Now try breathing in for 4-counts; out for 8-counts—slowly.
- *Another popular method:* Breathe in for 4-counts, hold for 7-counts, and breathe out for 8-counts—slowly.

Remember, every breath means you are still alive and that the most important part of your life is still ahead of you.

Soma (Body) Relaxation
- Sit comfortably or lie on the floor. Close your eyes.
- Flex and tighten your feet for two seconds while inhaling deeply.
- Hold your breath and then exhale deeply.
- Relax your tightened muscles after each deep exhale.
- Do this with all your muscle groups: the calves, buttocks, stomach, hands, shoulders, face, scalp and ears.

Appendix C

WARNING SIGNS OF AN UNHEALTHY AND ABUSIVE RELATIONSHIP

Toxic people attach themselves like cinder blocks tied to your ankles, and then invite you for a swim in their poisoned waters. —John Mark Green

Like a magnet, I (Kimberly) was constantly drawn to the "wrong kind of guy." It was always "infatuation at first sight." I didn't spend much time getting to know the person I was dating or potentially marrying. It didn't cross my mind to ask: *Does his personal information check out? Does he really work where he says he does? Has he been married before? Why did he get divorced? Can I meet his family?* I spent more time researching which new appliance or car to buy.

Just as there are serial abusers, so are there serial victims—women who continue to select multiple abusive partners. We're in this good healthy place now and need to stay this way, which means choosing to hang out with and date healthy people. Like they say, if it looks too good, take caution because it could be rotten inside.

Relationship experts say, the more deeply involved we become with a controlling, intimidating, or manipulative person, the more difficult to get out of the relationship. Then we find we're spiraling out of control again.

Domestic abuse is committed by people who are often described as being the sweetest, kindest, gentlest persons in the world. It's true. We say, "I can't imagine he'd hurt me." If you can't imagine it, then you won't see the warning signs. They may behave this way in the beginning, but there are always red flags. God says to *"live wisely"* (Colossians 4:5). The following list of warning signs could mean the start of an unhealthy and/or abusive relationship. If the signs are there, act quickly to either set strong boundaries or get out of the relationship. This red flag list also applies to friendships.

A push for quick involvement. This is when a person comes on really strong. He pressures you to be his wife/girlfriend immediately. He uses the word "we" prematurely (you and he are a team or couple); gives unsolicited promises.

Ignoring the word "no" is a signal that someone is either seeking control or refusing to relinquish it. If you let him talk you out of the word no, then you are saying, "I'm not in charge."

Overly charming and nice. There is often a motive behind this behavior. Gavin DeBecker said to think of charm as a verb, not a trait. If you tell yourself, "This person is trying to charm me," as opposed to "This person is charming," you'll be on guard to any deception. Niceness doesn't necessarily mean goodness.

Lack of trust. Does he not like you to go out with others without him? Does he read your texts and/or mail? You should be able to trust your partner not to cheat or poke around or spy.

I've learned as a counselor that apart from knowing someone well for many years, there is no foolproof rule or test for trustworthiness. When it comes to trusting other people, we all make mistakes. The bad news is there is 10% of the population that have no conscience and cannot be trusted. The good news is at least 90% can be counted on to behave according to a reasonably high baseline of decency and responsibility.

Frequently insulting. Does your relationship consist of constant criticism? Do you feel like you always have to be on the defense? Does he have a negative or condescending attitude about women; enjoy "pushing your buttons;" say mean, hurtful things; degrade, curse, or call you ugly names? Another sign would be *no* communication; and/or changes in mood or behavior. The person who loves you should make you feel spectacular, and not be constantly putting you down.

Is self-centered. Does he spend most of your time together talking. Does he shift the conversation to himself and not listen intently when you speak? Does he say "trust me!" a lot?

Lack of respect. Many men have stereotyped beliefs about women's roles. Does he frequently break promises or criticize or is rude to you? Does he speak disrespectfully about former partners? If yes, he won't hold you up in high esteem. No child of God should have to feel put down or feel like they're not valued. Disrespect can also take the form of *idealizing and worshipping* you—you're a fantasy or object.

Regularly picks a fight. Every relationship has its bumps, but if you're constantly fighting, particularly over small things, and you're frequently being picked at or bullied, this is a warning sign. The good days should outweigh the bad ones, not the other way around. When he resolves conflict, is it with TIME (threat, intimidation, manipulation, escalation)?

There is abuse. Does he threaten you with physical or sexual abuse/violence? Does he minimize incidents of abuse? Has he killed or harmed an animal? This is a *big* warning you're in a relationship with an unhealthy person.

Intimidates when offended. Does he get too close, put a finger in your face, poke or push, block or restrain you when he's mad? Does he raise a fist, tower over you, drive recklessly, or throw things around, or destroy property when he's annoyed or mad? Does he deny he's being aggressive? Danger sign!

Social isolation. Does he try to keep you from spending time with your family and friends? We need our families and friends. We need others' opinions besides our mate's. If you find that he expects you to only spend time with him, this is a red flag.

Always blaming. Does he blame you for problems or mistakes? This type of person doesn't take responsibility for their mistakes. Instead, it's always another person's fault.

Lies or omits the truth. A person might not exactly be lying about something, but they aren't telling the truth either. While you don't necessarily need to tell him "everything," each person should be equally open with the other person.

Truth is fundamental and foundational to all relationships. Relationships dissolve for lack of truth. (Truth is also foundational to our relationship with God.) DeBecker said that when people lie, even if what they say sounds credible to you, it doesn't sound credible to them so they *keep talking*. Be wary of too many details. Dr. Martha Stout suggests making the "Rule of Threes" a personal policy. One lie or broken promise may be a misunderstanding. Two is a serious mistake. But three lies say we're dealing with a deceitful liar.

Attempts to control. We all appreciate being able to go to our boyfriend/ husband to get advice but, if he continually advises or influences you to do certain things, it can be an attempt to control you. Does he tell you who to be friends with, what to wear, what to buy, or what to do with your time? Does he feel he has the right to know where you are all the time? Red flags!

Keeps secrets. In a healthy relationship, couples should be able to talk openly with one another without having to keep secrets.

Pressures for sex. A person who loves and respects their partner doesn't push them to have sex. They don't make the other person feel they owe it to them. Consider this viewpoint: When someone can say no to sex while dating, their behavior is a sign that he or she is capable of delaying gratification and exhibiting self-control, which are two prerequisites of the ability to love. If someone cannot delay gratification and control himself in this area, most likely they cannot delay their own gratification in other areas of sacrifice.

Unhealthy jealousy and possessiveness. Does he keep tabs on you; feel anxious about your associations with other men, especially ex-partners? Does he expect you to give up your freedom for him and be "together for life"? Does he compete with your friends? Is he envious of something you have or do? He should be happy for you and your accomplishments, and not competing.

No compromise. The key of any relationship is the ability to compromise. We can't always have things go exactly the way we want. If he isn't able to make allowances for you, it will make your life and relationship very difficult.

Loves being in love. Might he "be in love with being in love" (but he's not really in love)? Has he gotten serious too quickly? He may have come to believe that not having a romantic relationship means there's something wrong with him. He may feel that having a wife or girlfriend proves his worth or is his "trophy." Some feel a bad or violent relationship is better than no relationship at all. They won't ever be happy.

Frequently plays for your pity or flatters you in an extreme way. This is a mark of a sociopath.[138]

Confuses you regularly. Abuse experts say that the one most common negative effect abusers cause above all others is *confusion:* if you spend a lot of time feeling baffled by what is going on and stressed about what will come next.[139] Also be aware of inconsistent and confusing stories.

According to behavioral specialist Gavin DeBecker, some other red flags are:

- Uses alcohol or drugs with adverse effects like hostility, cruelty, or memory loss.
- History of police encounters.
- Uses "male privilege" to justify his behavior.
- Refuses to accept rejection; Dark humor.
- Paranoid: believes others are out to get him.
- Resists change; is inflexible, unwilling to compromise.
- Sees weapons as instruments of power, control or revenge.
- History of childhood abuse or witnessing violence as a kid.
- Speaks only of his "potential." For example, *I'm not working now but I'll be really successful; I'm going to be a great painter but can't under these circumstances; The reason I'm acting this way is I'm on edge until I get settled.*

No single one of these warning signs is a sure sign of an unhealthy or abusive man, except for abuse and control. Healthy men may have some of these behaviors to a limited degree. Make it clear which behaviors and attitudes are unacceptable. Set every boundary with a consequence.

For example, *"I can't be in a relationship with you if you continue to [name behavior]. … If you don't stop doing this, I'll have to terminate our relationship."* Stick to your consequence! If you give him too many chances, you're likely to regret it. If he switches to another red flag behavior, chances are he has a problem—*get out.*

Bottom line: *Trust your gut—your survival instinct.* It's a gift from God. It's always in response to something, and always has your best interests at heart. It's the Holy Spirit speaking to you and trying to protect you. Listen for: nagging feelings, fear, anxiety, suspicion and apprehension, gut feelings, persistent thoughts, curiosity, hunches, doubt and hesitation. Never stay when you really want out.

Lastly, spend at least one year getting to know the person before making any major commitments. If the relationship feels too intense, like it's going to fast, or you're feeling disrespected or uncomfortable with his expectations, then listen to your gut. *See what other wise people think.* Ask for their honest feedback and listen to them.

Guys Who Can't Let Go (Getting Rid of Mr. Wrong)

Have you noticed in our culture that men who pursue unlikely or inappropriate relationships with women, and then get them, is a common theme? The Hollywood formula is: *Boy wants girl. Girl doesn't want boy. Boy harasses girl. Boy gets girl.* This harassment is disguised under "playing hard to get," or "She really wanted me all along but needed to realize it."

In other words, "no" is not what she really meant. Really? In Hollywood, when men pursue, they usually get the girl; when women pursue, she usually gets killed.

Stalking is how some guys raise the stakes when the woman won't play along. It's a crime of power, control and intimidation through persistent phone calls and messages; showing up uninvited; following her; trying to engage her friends or family in his agenda, for example.

An unwanted pursuer (stalker) inadvertently is saying, "You aren't allowed to decide who will be in your life." They are the kind of people that don't give up easily and don't let go. Guys who can't let go typically choose women who can't say no. If you criticize and rudely tell him to get lost you may find he's very sensitive to rejection and will interpret your actions as insulting or threatening. If you take him on, you can become his "target."

How do we get rid of Mr. Wrong? Again, I look to the counsel of expert Gavin DeBecker who asserts there is one rule: *Do not negotiate. Stop all contact.* Once a woman makes the decision, she doesn't want a relationship with a particular man, it needs to be said *one time—explicitly*. Almost any contact after that rejection will be seen as a negotiation.

If a woman repeatedly tells a guy she doesn't want to talk to him, that is talking to him. And every time she does, she is further away from resolving the matter. Her actions must match her words. *Any response is progress to him.* Don't get trapped in the "It's not very Christian to treat a fellow human, or believer, this way." Setting boundaries in order to protect your safety and well-being is biblical.

When a woman gets 30 messages from a pursuer and doesn't call him back, but then finally gives in and returns his calls (*He seemed so nice and enthusiastic*), he learns that the cost of reaching her is leaving 30 messages. When we reject someone and say something like, "I just don't want to be in a relationship right now," he hears, "Maybe later." Get the point?

DeBecker suggests that women never explain why they don't want a relationship, but simply make it clear that it is their decision and they expect the guy to accept and respect it. A rejection based on any condition or excuse gives him something to challenge.

Remember: The best response is *no response*. Here's a classic line in DeBecker's book, "*The fact that a romantic pursuer is relentless doesn't mean you are special—it means he is troubled.*"

These guys are essentially "detoxing" from their addiction to love and the relationship. The difference is in a stalking case it is usually one-sided; the stalker is the addict and his object of affection is the drug. Small doses of the drug (you) won't wean him off. As with most addictions, abstinence and cold turkey, which means no contact, is the solution.

Note on *restraining orders:* Victims of stalkers get the same advice given to battered women—get a restraining order. As with battered women, it's important to evaluate whether the situation might be improved or worsened by court intervention. Pray and seek wisdom from the Holy Spirit.

Dating carries several risks: the risk of disappointment, of rejection, and the risk of letting some troubled guy into your life. Once again, to avoid these situations, listen to your gut (the Holy Spirit) right from the get go—and your good friends' gut. First Peter 5:8 says, "*Be sober-minded; be watchful. Your adversary the devil prowls around like a roaring lion, seeking someone to devour.*"

† If you're trying to get rid of Mr. Wrong, would you say your actions are matching your words?

What Your Body Language Says

Abusers and con artists have a special kind of antennae that picks up the frequency of potential victims. They seem know from a woman's posture and gait who would be a good target. They may lack the capacity to empathize and read emotions, yet their predatory ability to read fear and helplessness is expertly honed. They seem to be able to look into a person's eyes and spot the vulnerable.

Do you want to resolve the fear of future adversity? You can by learning to be smart and walk with purpose in a confident way that reduces your risk of being taken advantage of. You can start right now by visualizing yourself projecting strong body language.

In a classic study, researchers Betty Grayson and Morris Stein asked convicted criminals to view a video of pedestrians walking down a busy New York City sidewalk. There was a clear consensus among the criminals about whom they would have picked as victims—and their choices were not based on gender, race, or age. For example, some petite women were not selected as potential victims, while some large men were.

The criminals assessed which people they could overpower based on several nonverbal signals—*posture, body language, pace of walking, length of stride,* and *awareness of environment.* Perpetrators notice a person whose *walk* lacks organized movement and flowing motion—perhaps because their walk suggests they are less athletic and fit. They view such people as *less self-confident* and are much more likely to exploit them.

Sexual predators in particular look for people they can easily overpower. A convicted sex offender who raped 75 women said, "If I had an inkling that a woman wasn't someone I could easily handle, then I'd pass right on by. Or if I thought I couldn't control the situation, I wouldn't even mess with the house, or attempt a rape there."

Criminologist, Tod Burke, said, "The rapist is going to go after somebody who's not paying attention, who looks like they're not going to put up a fight, who's in a location that's going to make this more convenient."

Rapists tend to be able to interpret facial cues, such as a downward gaze or a fearful expression, suggestive of submissive women. Speaking of rape: Safety experts agree that there are no cookie-cutter answers. For example, some say if you're raped do not resist; others say to resist. Neither strategy is wrong or right, but one strategy is—listen to your intuition which is collecting all the information.

Distraction is another cue. Some people think talking on a cell phone enhances their safety because the other person can always summon help if there's trouble, but experts disagree. Talking or texting on any device is a distraction, and predators are looking for distracted victims.

Ex-FBI and behavioral specialist, Joe Navarro, speaking of women's body language, said, "Standing with their feet together (which is perceived as submissive) sends the wrong kind of signal to a would-be antagonist. By moving their feet apart, females can take a more dominant, "I am in charge," stance."[140]

Passive and permissive personalities are most likely to be assaulted. If a woman convincingly yells, "Stop!"—marking a strong and clear boundary, they're more likely to leave her alone. Predatory men can accurately identify submissive women by their style of dress and other aspects of appearance. The hallmarks of submissive body language, such as downward gaze and slumped posture, may even be misinterpreted by rapists as flirtation.

Interpersonal violence increases between the hours of 8:00 pm and 2 am. Criminologist, Kim Rossmo, found that great white sharks and serial killers have common behavioral traits, in terms of how they hunt their prey. They are both focused killers, prefer their victims to be young and alone, and like to attack when the light is low.[141]

The woman who jogs and enjoys listening to music through earbuds has disabled her hearing—a sense most likely to warn her against danger. Drinking and drug use mark a person. Drunken people appear more vulnerable and are likely to put themselves in dangerous situations. Women who are intoxicated, studies confirm, tend to be animated, giving off signals sexual offenders may misinterpret as sexual interest.

Stay aware of your surroundings at all times and avoid dangerous situations. Criminals prefer sites that serve up few witnesses and little chance of being caught. If you see a person walking around with seemingly no purpose, who suddenly makes a beeline for you, be aware. If you speak with a stranger whose nose begins flaring, experts say this is suspicious behavior.[142] Many women choose to take a self-defense class to learn skills to help prevent and interrupt an attack and heal from past abuse by feeling empowered and strong.

I would add, when walking in unfamiliar territory keep your hands out of your pockets. If you have to run, and you fall, your arms won't be able to cushion your fall. There's a good chance you'll land on your beautiful face and break your nose and/or teeth.

By using our bodies differently, we can create greater confidence and move forward when we feel afraid. When people breathe deeply, lift their chest, move their shoulders back, and keep their head up, and walk with purpose, this power pose says, "I'm not just another person walking on the street. Watch out!" Always listen to your inner voice and remember—you're the daughter of God. No one has any right to mess with you!

Protecting Ourselves

A man with conviction is a hard man to change. –Leon Festinger, PhD

Dangerous personalities are all around us—and that is why we have to be particularly on guard. –Joe Navarro, ex-FBI Behavioral specialist

There are things we can do every day, experts say, to protect ourselves and our children. In a nutshell, we need to:

- *Gain knowledge.* This book is a beginning point. There are many good books and websites out on this subject.
- *Become an observer.* People today have their faces buried in their smartphones; they don't observe. Predators know this!
- *Distance yourself.* If someone is wearing you down, or trying to control your space, put up a barrier and distance yourself. Set boundaries and walk away.
- *Don't wait too long to act.* If you sense something isn't right, act on it.
- *Trust your gut and the Holy Spirit's promptings.* Gavin de Becker wrote, "Trust your intuition (rather than technology) to protect you from violence ... it's the exact opposite of living in fear ... and never show fear." I say pray for wisdom and discernment regarding your situation. If your gut says to cut the emotional strings and the relationship, do it.

We also need to know if this person is dangerous. Let's see what the experts say. The more yes answers to these questions, the more likely you're dealing with someone who has traits of a dangerous personality.[143]

- Do they affect you emotionally in a negative way?
- Do they do things that are illegal, erratic, unethical, or defy social norms, or are dangerous??
- Do they do things that are abusive or manipulative?
- Do they do things impulsively with little control or with unwillingness to delay gratification?

How many yeses did you count? Two or more? Take Dr. Henry Cloud's advice, "Tell him or her goodbye and save yourself a lot of heartache ... no matter how much you are attracted to him or her. Run, run, run!" Let go of the optimistic and false image you had of the person you loved. Sadly, that person never existed. He (or she) was only an illusion, a mask the abuser created in order control and manipulate you.

Remember this: *The abuses committed against us, whether physical, sexual, verbal, or emotional, are not our sins.* Those sins belong to the offender/abuser. Despite what your abuser, or a person covering for the abuser, may have told you, *you did not deserve the abuse, or do anything to warrant it. You're not responsible.* Let me also say, anyone has the right to question authority.

Lastly, many victims ask for couple's counseling. The abuser may finally agree to go when the victim is serious about leaving him. *Couples counseling is not recommended for many reasons, particularly if there is violence, or power and control tactics being used.* Counseling can take place *after* he has worked through his power and control issues. He must display genuine repentance, accountability, and a new pattern of relating.

Hope for a Future
Let me assure you—life exists on the other side. Everyone grieves differently. Every person has a different recovery time. On the average, it takes a good year to get your heart into a good place. With time, and relying on God and His power and wisdom, you will begin to find moments of joy, contentment, and hope for a future.

When our hearts and minds focus on the things of God, and when our spirits, no matter how damaged, are united with God's Spirit, we can feel safe, ready to express ourselves, and move forward.

Letting go of the "dream man" will bring you closer to Jesus—your real Prince, and your real self. We will likely encounter toxic people in the future. As we connect with God and other kind, loving, and passionate people, a newfound strength will merge.

† Describe how equipped emotionally, physically, and spiritually you feel in regards to starting your life over. Name what can you accept/not accept?

Appendix D

PROFILE OF AN ABUSER & PREDATOR

> *... they loved the darkness [sin] more than the Light [God], for their deeds were evil.* –Jesus, speaking John 3:19

> *Important: I don't work with abusers. Yet, I want to share with you what I have learned. The material is intended to validate and affirm that you're not alone—nor crazy! This material is not meant to be used for diagnostic purposes. Please handle it with care. I don't intend for the information to be used to harm or destroy anyone. We're not criminologists or profilers. Abusers and predators are themselves deceived. Yet, when a person will not admit their sin, and becomes dangerous and violent, then action must be taken. Vigilance and knowledge will keep us and our children safe. In the end, we must rely on our distinctive abilities to sense danger. We ask the Lord to heighten our powers of observation. If you start to feel overwhelmed or triggered, step away. Pray and apply the self-care deep breathing exercises in Appendix B.*

"**K**imberly, there's a guy I want you to meet. His name is Bill and I think you guys will hit it off. He's charming and adorable. You'll love him!" As you will recall from my account in *Loving Someone with a Personality Disorder (chapter 13)*, unbeknownst to me, I fell into a relationship with a predator.

The "Romantic" Play Begins

> *An abuser's behavior is primarily conscious—he acts deliberately rather than by accident or by losing control of himself—but the underlying thinking that drives his behavior is largely not conscious.* –Lundy Bancroft, Why Does He Do That?

After being introduced to Bill, he immediately "love-bombed" me with flattery and attention. "Kim, I can tell you're going to be very easy to fall in love with." I turned to mush. He led me to believe I won "the prize," that many women were dying to date him. He had skillfully manufactured the illusion of being popular by surrounding himself with friends and former exes. I did believe I won the prize. (Whether accurate or not, we're usually quite confident in our first impressions.)

The high level of attention he paid to me felt so good. We created a very quick emotional and physical bond. We partied and drank alcohol a lot. From that point on we were almost inseparable. One month later, Bill asked me to marry him. He moved into my condo and agreed to pay half my mortgage and utilities … and he asked me to charge my engagement ring to my credit card, promising to pay me back.

He had a plan: to latch on to me and steal what I worked hard to attain. Some professionals call this "economic exploitation." He also had a young child from a previous marriage who he didn't tell me about initially and didn't support (red flag!).

The Abuse Heightens
Not long after, things changed. He never paid me a dime for anything. I noticed my credit cards disappeared and reappeared. He'd forgo plans he made with me, and didn't come home many nights, claiming he went out drinking with friends and couldn't drive home.

Bill was a gaslighter. He'd make unfounded accusations. One morning I told him I was meeting Sharon after work. Sharon cancelled so I invited another friend, Monica. (Monica was the ex of his boss, whom he now disliked. We'd all hung out in the recent past). Screaming, he accused me of purposefully lying to him about meeting Monica. I told him repeatedly what had transpired. The truth didn't matter. In his mind, I was supposed to be listening and agreeing with him, not arguing. He got so teed-off at "my lying" that he punched a hole into the wall, then stomped out and didn't return until the next day. Like so many previous times before, I just wanted to be heard, but he never heard me. To him, I had no voice.

Trying to defend myself from false accusations was not uncommon. Bill only saw it as criticism, and then he'd turn on me with anger. My love transformed into anxiety, crying, and sleepless nights. Some days I felt insane, exhausted, shocked, and empty—all the while he enjoyed manipulating me. It was hard to avoid explosive situations. It was exhausting living with him. But I never once wondered if this was abuse.

(Many experts agree that abusers carry attitudes that produce anger and rage—*but anger is not the cause of abuse*. Abusers aren't abusive because they're mad. Professionals say it does little good to send them to an anger management program because their sense of entitlements keep producing more anger. Their *attitudes and beliefs* are what must change.)

Bill subtly imposed his system on me which exempted him from society's rules and standards. The rules applied to me, but not him. For example, he allowed himself to have occasional affairs because "men have their needs." If I were to have an affair, who knows what horrible thing he'd have done. He argued and yelled constantly. If I yelled back, I was "a hysterical woman." He didn't need to account for his time because he was "the man," but I did.

Breaking Up

The most heartbreaking moment came when Bill broke the engagement and moved into a house with a friend. (I should have been ecstatic!) He vowed he still loved me and wanted to continue to date. The problem was, while I desperately tried to repair our relationship, he'd already started another one.

I loved him so much that I accepted the deal because I naively believed things would change. Even though I had "knowledge of good and evil" I chose to continue to tolerate toxic behavior. Renowned criminologist Dr. Leonard Territo described women like me as "victims in search of an oppressor."[144] I couldn't help but wonder what I did wrong; what my personal deficits were that drove him away. I realize now I was "trauma-bonded" to Bill. I had a hard time letting go of my dream—a wonderful marriage with kids and the perfect man.

Putting the Puzzle Pieces Together

How much time have you wasted trying to figure out what is wrong with you, rather than what is wrong with your abusive partner? Probably a lot! These guys put on a charming face for the outside world, creating a sharp split between their public and their home image. Lundy Bancroft stated, "One of the obstacles to recognizing chronic mistreatment is that most abusive men simply don't *seem* like abusers. ... These men usually keep their abusive side well-hidden outside of the home."[145]

The day came when I finally grasped Bill was a narcissistic con man, and I'd been brainwashed. Everything started to fall into place. God gave me the backbone to finally stand up to him and say, "No more!"

- I recognized the urgency to detach from this toxic relationship, and that as a child of God I didn't have to endure bad relationships.
- I didn't let him make me feel guilty, nor explain myself to him.
- I felt it was better to be alone than in a destructive relationship.
- I knew I had to take care of myself. *It's my life to live!*

I never saw him again. Halleluiah! Apparently, Bill was untouched. He just went on to his next victim. Healing began when I realized all the insecurities I had were manufactured by him. As I look back on this pain-filled 18-months (seemed like 10 years), Bill offered absolutely nothing of value to our relationship—only false praise and insincere flattery. Before Bill came into my life, I had a steady job, friends, and normal insecurities. After he was done with me, my life was destroyed. I lost my job and good friends, was depressed and anxious, and consumed with mind-boggling insecurities.

What I learned was *this is how abused people feel—but this was not the real me. There was nothing wrong with me. I did nothing wrong. His abuse tactics were his problem, not mine.* Bill was abused as a child and his desire was to control everything from that point forward. Mind control was the name of the game. Because he couldn't control the mind of his abuser, it became his goal to control the minds of those he violated.

> *You never have to tolerate being hurt by anyone. If you are being abused by your partner, you can call the National Domestic Hotline at 800-799-7233; National Resource Center on Domestic Violence at 800-537-2238. Pray and seek wise counsel!*

The Aftermath of Love and War

"Why me?" How many *"If only I hadn't ... If only I had ...* statements have you verbalized? "How could I have been so gullible, letting him hijack my free will? The fact is: Bill set a trap; I unknowingly ate the toxic bait. But—this doesn't mean I'm crazy or stupid.

Don't beat yourself up. You didn't voluntarily form a bond with a betrayer. Your consent was based on a lie. It's not your fault. You were tricked into feeling an overwhelming strong attachment during the dating "grooming" period. You weren't targeted because you were stupid or 'less than.' On the contrary, you were probably targeted for the many good qualities you possess.

You never expected to enter a love relationship expecting to be manipulated, abused, belittled, and criticized, did you? Me either. I was tricked into falling in love, which is hard to resist considering it's the strongest human emotion. Let's not forget, this was never God's blueprint for a man-woman relationship As the Bible says, *"God is not a God of disorder but of peace"* (1 Corinthians 14:33). And, *"for Satan himself masquerades as an angel of light"* (2 Corinthians 11:14).

If you were replaced by another woman, there's nothing wrong with you. You've been created by God Almighty "very good" (Genesis 1:31). The person who treated you so badly is not capable of loving another human being the way God designed love. *There's nothing you could have done differently.*

Now you know the truth. You haven't lost everything. You've gained everything—you just don't realize it yet. You can break free from these traps. God can use your desire for change and justice to your advantage.

The Mystery of an Abusive Mate

Dating an emotional predator, such as a narcissist or sociopath, or anyone else who has the potential to be abusive or toxic is a devastating emotional roller coaster of highs and lows—of high conflict. They tend to reveal their true selves after they've already reeled their victims in. My goal is to give you some real-life information and some key signs to look out.

According to Retired FBI Special Agent, Joe Navarro, author of *Dangerous Personalities,* these guys "have only one goal: exploitation. They live to plunder, rob, victimize, or destroy. ... These individuals don't think as we do. We care about others. They pretend to care or simply don't. ... They use words to manipulate, compel, and connive ... For many predators, it's about the godlike ability to have power over others, which can be intoxicating ... If you survive one of these individuals, a part of you dies—be it trust, self-worth, dignity, or faith in others."

If you now recognize you've been attached to one of these guys, listen to what Dr. Robert Hare, the creator of the standard diagnostic *Psychopathy Checklist,* wrote: "Everyone, including experts, can be taken in, manipulated, conned, and left bewildered by them. A good psychopath can play a concerto on *anyone's* heartstrings ... Your best defense is to understand the nature of these human predators."

According to Lundy Bancroft, *Why Does He Do That*

> The abuser's mood changes are especially perplexing. He can be a different person from day to day, even hour to hour. Like Rambo, at times, he is aggressive and intimidating, his tone harsh, insults spewing from his mouth, ridicule dripping from him like oil from a drum. When he's in this mode, nothing she says seems to have any impact, except to make him angrier. Her side of the argument counts for nothing in his eyes, and everything is her fault. He twists her words around so that she always ends up on the defensive.

At other moments, he sounds wounded and lost, hungering for love and for someone to take care of him. When this side of him emerges, he appears open and ready to heal. He seems to let down his guard, his hard exterior softens, and he may take on the quality of a hurt child, difficult and frustrating but lovable. Looking at him in this deflated state, his partner has trouble imagining that the abuser inside of him will ever be back. The beast that takes him over at other times looks completely unrelated to the tender person she now sees. Sooner or later, though, the shadow comes back over him, as if it had a life of its own.[146]

We have a hard time believing this "great guy" is a predator because we feel confident in our abilities to detect a lie. Their kind of deception is hard for most people to accept. It means that someone whom we like and trust has been conning us. Don't feel stupid, police officers and judges and psychiatrists can only spot a liar 50% of the time.

The abusive person is a mystery. While they don't dress or appear any differently, they may be recognized if we choose to remove our blinders. A parent or woman's false sense of confidence regarding their ability to pick out an abuser, is a reason why predators are able to victimize so many children and women. You can protect yourself from becoming a victim by vaccinating yourself with as much knowledge as possible, and you'll be in a better position to protect your loved ones. Recognizing the nature of an abuser can be the first step out of the fog. There is no single profile, but there are distinguishable characteristics abusers share.

Characteristics of An Abusive Person

> *Little is known about the mind of the abuser. Since he is disapproving of those who seek to understand him, he does not volunteer to be studied. Since he does not perceive that anything is wrong with him, he does not seek help—unless he is in trouble with the law. ... How much more comforting it would be if the abuser were easily recognizable.* –Judith Herman, M.D.

One day, Tanya told Danny that his outbursts were getting to her, and she wanted to take a time-out from their relationship. Danny got right into her face and said, "You're saying that you don't love me anymore! You probably never loved me. You have no idea how much I love you!" The conversation then shifted. Tanya reassured Danny that she wasn't abandoning him.

Then Tanya told Danny she wanted to go back to school. He responded negatively, "We can't afford it and I'm not going to take care of the baby." Tanya then proposed some strategies—all of which Danny found something wrong with. So, Tanya decided the time was not right to pursue her education. Danny insists he wasn't trying to talk her out of it. She believes her decision was her own.

Why did Danny use intimidation and manipulation to control her? He found Tanya's taking a class threatening to his control over her. Abusers are uncomfortable when they see signs of independence in their partners, so will find ways to undermine their progress.

They are pros at getting the victim to believe she has unreasonable expectations and she is reacting to something in her life, not to what he did. His toxic behavior gets pointed back to the victim. They seem to share unique aspects to their personalities. (Shame is most likely to be the cause of these behaviors.)

Common characteristics are:

Betray—lure through a promise or expectation; read their victims well by appealing to their desolation or woundedness.

Intimidate—through anger and manipulation. Many use physical threats or violence as an intimidation tactic.

Selfish—caring more about themselves than others. When an abusive guy focuses on his partner, most of what he thinks about is what she can do for him, not the other way around. He confuses love with lust.

Narcissistic & emotionally unstable personality—an egotistical cover for an inferiority complex which compels them to strive for superiority: "Nothing is more important to me than me. I have no empathy for you. And I am *always* right; you are wrong." Not sure if you're with a narcissist? When was the last time he asked you how *you felt* about something?

Unable to experience complicated emotions like shame and guilt, or love and joy.

Paranoid—is deeply *suspicious* and constantly *fears* betrayal. Because they imagine conspiracies against them, they will launch preemptive attacks against their targets (victims), hoping to hurt them first. They bear grudges for minor or nonexistent reasons. For example, they may suspect you are having affairs, hiding money, or lying to them about something.

Abrupt mood shifts which last for short periods. If you've ever been in a relationship that was highly charged and generally short-lived, where the person frantically pursues and needs you one minute, then sends you packing the next; is filled with turbulence and rage one day, then wonder and excitement the next—you may be with a person who is "borderline," short for *Borderline Personality Disorder (BPD)*.[147]

Control others feelings, thoughts, and behaviors through empty promises and lying; bullying and threats, pleading and begging; crying, sulking, acting despondent and dependent, withdrawing, even threatening suicide.

For example, an abusive husband may consider it his right to tell his wife where to go, what to wear, whom to associate with, and when she needs to be home. Many are what we'd call a "Drill Sergeant." They leave you feeling troubled, unfulfilled, and tormented.

Lack of accountability. They think they're above the law; above criticism. They believe they should be allowed to ignore the damage their behavior is causing—and may even retaliate if anyone gets them to look at it. In the effort to be free from accountability, they focus on their partner's faults.

Blames others to avoid accepting responsibility and admitting they did something wrong. To him, *you* are the cause of his behavior. For example, a rapist may say the victim wanted sex by the way she dressed or acted. This makes him feel stronger, creating a false sense of safety. They use "you" statements: "You made me hit you."

Abusers condition their victims to believe the problem isn't the abuse itself, it's *your reaction* to the abuse—that's the problem. They're pros at *minimizing*. They compare their actions to others who do worst things and conclude they're not abusive. In the end, the abuser is responsible to God for what he does. Blame won't cut it.

View themselves as victims no matter how horribly they've treated someone. They even adopt the same language as abuse victims. Since nothing is ever their fault, they're the ones who've been wronged. Everything revolves around their woundedness. If you feel sorry for him, then he can remain the center of attention.

Judges others by being extremely critical. They're dismissive and judgmental if you try to disprove their story. You may develop perfectionist qualities, aware that any mistake will be used against you.

Jealous and possessive. Accusations of flirting and cheating are common, even though abusers are most likely to be cheating themselves. Extreme jealousy is exhibited though a desire to isolate the partner from any source of emotional support, information or aid. Then she can be totally focused on his needs and desires.

He also doesn't want her to develop sources of strength which could lead to her independence. A common theory is: Abusers have a fear of abandonment. (Post-separation homicides of intimate partners are committed almost exclusively by men. There is usually a history of abuse *before* the breakup.[148])

Gaslights: they use manipulation or "crazy making" tactics such as changing their moods, voice tone, and facial features abruptly and frequently; get you to feel sorry for him and/or blame yourself for what he does; uses confusion tactics; lies and misleads to get what he wants; messes up her relationships by lying, betraying confidences and other divisive tactics.[149] *Denial* is common. These people know exactly how to get under your skin. They can easily convince other people that we're the messed-up ones.

Deceives others by manipulating words and actions to confuse the victim and put her on the defense. They lie and have an excuse for everything. For example, they take your words, even Scripture, completely out of context. 1 Timothy 4:2 says, *"These liars have lied so well and for so long that they've lost their capacity for truth"* (MSG).

Use pity and sympathy. The battered wife whose husband moans that he can't control himself; that he's a poor wretch whom she must to forgive.

Offers compliments. What do you notice about these compliments?

- My ex and I always fought. You and I never fight.
- My ex always wanted to talk on the phone. I'm so glad you're not needy or demanding.
- My ex always nagged me about getting a job. You're so much more understanding.

These are not compliments; they are expectations. Each guy has come up with a list of traits that bother them. Then they plant the ideas in their partner's mind, which is manipulation. In other words, "Don't express or do these things (fight, want to talk on the phone, or nag) or else." He convinces you that what *he* wants you to do is in *your* best interest.

Punishment is a retaliation tactic for resisting their control or speaking truth.

Entitlement is the belief they have a special status which gives them exclusive rights and privileges that don't apply to their partner. For example, they can have an affair, but not their partner. Or, they feel entitled to forgiveness. *My partner should be grateful I apologized!*

Projects onto others. If they can shift the focus from themselves onto others, then they won't be called out for their bad behavior. It's "Shame on *you*!"

Sexual manipulation means the abuser considers it his partner's duty to keep him sexually satisfied; he feels entitled to do as he pleases. Passionate sex marks the beginning of the relationship. Then he begins playing games: withholding sex, redefining it as a privilege, and making specific demands.
    Forced or coerced sexual activity by a partner is sexual assault. Partner rape is real rape. Partner rape is a crime of violence more than a crime of passion. These men want to control, and they use sex as their weapon of choice. After the rape, they feel more powerful and in control. Yet, the woman is vulnerable to trauma. This is because the person she'd normally run to for protection is her source of danger. Therefore, professional help is advised so she can rebuild a sense of control and trust in future sexual relations.

The "Normal" Abuser

> *Sometimes he's so nice and charming. He goes to church a lot, and everyone thinks he's wonderful. They just don't know the side I see at home. It's like he's Dr. Jekyll and Mr. Hyde.* –Aimee

Do you relate to what Aimee is saying? Nobody really has any idea who the "real" guy is. The thing about an abusive relationship is it's not so obvious. You don't understand you're in one until you're in too deep or long after it's over. Eventually you see a side of him that never came out during the dating and honeymoon phase—the cold, inconsiderate, and manipulative side. "What happened to the person I fell in love with?" *What happened?*

What I've learned in studying profiles of abusive people is that the great majority of them would be deemed psychologically normal. Their minds work logically, they understand cause and effect, and they don't hallucinate. *Their value system is unhealthy, not necessarily their psychology and brain. Generally speaking, most abusers are not psychopaths.*

Beliefs, values, and habits govern abusive or controlling behavior. Most have a conscience about their behavior outside of home. They are willing to be accountable. Even when mental illness or addiction is a factor, it *is not the cause*. It does nevertheless contribute to the severity of the abuse and resistance to change.[150]

Abusers desire to dominate their partners sexually, emotionally, and physically. They thrive on creating confusion and do this by exploiting our vulnerabilities. They don't necessarily use physical aggression to control, although sometimes they resort to it. Instead, they consume a person by manufacturing the *illusion* of love—and only leave pain, confusion, and chaos in their path of destruction.

I want to address the "don't talk" unspoken rule. If we've been violated and refuse to talk about it, not only will healing be obstructed, but then the offender will not be held accountable for his actions. If we let them continue with their behaviors without accountability, we are enhancing a system that is in opposition to the freedom that is in Christ.

Why Does He Do That?

How many times have you asked this most common question, *"Why does he (she) do that?"* This is what the experts believe: Abusiveness has less to do with psychological problems (such as personality disorders) and more to do with *values and beliefs*. Every person's values and beliefs grow out of:

- The family and home.
- Messages the child receive from toys and television.
- The neighborhood culture; peer groups.
- Training about sex roles and relationships.
- What we read, watch, hear, and see; media programming.
- Adult role models—personal and impersonal.
- Religious practices, or lack of.

David Sullivan wrote, "Nobody embraces false beliefs: we embrace something we think is true." Children are watching to see which behaviors get rewards and what makes a person popular, as opposed to those who are condemned to the outer circle. During the teen years, kids have access to the wider culture, with less filtering by parents and adults, and are subject to the influence of peer groups and the worship of celebrities.

Of all these influences, *the home is the greatest.* A boy who grows up in a home where Dad assaults Mom may observe that over the years Dad doesn't seem to get into serious trouble. He, therefore, views his dad's behavior as being acceptable. Add to this that culturally, legal consequences are less serious for men who assault their partners versus those who assault strangers. Boys often learn they're not responsible for their actions.

"The messages to young men, intentional or not, are that coercion and even a degree of physical violence and intimidation are compatible with deep love, and a man can know better than a woman what is good for her," stated Lundy Bancroft.

An abuser's values and beliefs develop from a range of cultural experiences. It's interesting because there may be other children in the abuser's family who don't abuse. It's like when one of your kids gets straight A's, and the other gets D's. Or, one child is in introvert; the other an extrovert. Where a kid will land on the abuse spectrum is also dependent on their personality type, personal predisposition, and birth order.

Be on Alert
- Listen to their *words* for threatening or extreme language.
- Check your own *emotions* for intense reactions. What do you feel around this person?
- Look for a history of high-conflict *behavior*. Has he/she acted in an extreme manner? Does he/she tend to blame others?

These people tend to do things that 90% of the population would never do. He said to ask ourselves, "Would 90% of the people (at work, in church, at a mall or stadium, etc.) do these things—"

- Hit a random stranger because they feel tired or stressed.
- Humiliate a friend in public because the person broke their trust.
- Destroy a child's favorite memento because the child broke a rule.
- Walk in front of a long line demanding to be waited on immediately because they are more important than the others.
- Gives someone an intense, intimate hug just after meeting them.
- Abruptly yell or go into a raging in a routine meeting or conversation.[151]
- Never ask, "What would *you* like?"

Judging Favorably

Many who regularly use power and control tactics do not intentionally set out to hurt and harm (yet, some do). Most are not inherently evil. They're often not even aware that their relational style is one of control, intimidation and manipulation. It's what has worked and what they know. Therefore, they see no reason to change. Many were born with a bent toward a personality disorder (genetics) or developed one because they were seriously abused or indulged in their childhoods (environment).

According to Dr. Bill Eddy, cofounder of the High Conflict Institute in San Diego, "their ability to be self-aware and change has been lost because of genetics and/or childhood environment, so they really cannot help themselves. They don't understand that they can improve by focusing on changing themselves instead of blaming others for their conflicts and emotions."[152]

Understand *you'll* never change an abuser, even when you confront their tactics directly; they'll probably switch tactics. They cannot change unless they overcome their core beliefs and values. Oswald Chambers wrote, "A child of the light will confess sin instantly and stand completely open before God. But a child of the darkness will say, "Oh, I can explain that."[153] We cannot change others. We can only change ourselves.

Do I Confront My Abuser?

I have heard from experts and victims that perpetrators rarely admit their actions. Some shrug it off as "no big deal." Others deny anything ever happened, or they've got a closet full of excuses.

If you ask the "why" questions and you don't get a satisfactory answer, then what do you get out of the confrontation? If you feel you must personally confront the person, please prepare yourself thoroughly.

- *You need to define the outcome you are seeking:* Is it an apology or reconciliation or forgiveness or a restriction?
- *Know exactly what you want to say.* Role play with someone else.
- *Remember: Your healing will not come from the abuser.*
- *Pick a safe place:* Choose a neutral location; bring someone else.
- *Be prepared to hear denials and excuses.*
- *Don't allow the abuser to get you off topic.*
- *Afterwards: De-brief and process with someone you can trust.*

Substance Addiction and Abusive Behavior

The role that alcohol, drugs, and other addictions play in abusive behavior is often misunderstood. Substance abuse is a misguided attempt to solve a problem. Most abusers who do abuse substances still mistreat their partners, even when they're not under the influence. It's been documented that abusers who successfully complete an addiction recovery program continue to abuse.

Yet, we do know alcohol and drug abuse can make matters worse. It tends to make the individual more unstable, less inhibited, and more dangerous. Alcohol encourages people to let loose what they've had simmering below the surface. Lundy Bancroft has counseled over 2000 abusive men. As an expert in this field, he is adamant,

> Addiction does not cause partner abuse, and recovery from addiction does not cure partner abuse. Alcohol does not directly make people belligerent, aggressive, or violent. Alcohol is a depressant, a substance that rarely causes aggression. Marijuana similarly has no biological action connected to abusiveness. Alcohol does not change a person's fundamental value system. People's conduct while intoxicated continue to be governed by their core foundation of beliefs and attitudes.[154]

While substance addiction does not *cause* a person to become abusive, it ensures the abusiveness *remains*. Substance abuse blocks the self-examination process. An abuser will most likely not make any significant changes in his behavior until he simultaneously deals with his substance abuse. These are two distinct problems which require two distinct solutions.

The same thing goes for *anger*. In attempting to repair the relationship, an abuser may say he couldn't help his rage; that he wasn't able to control himself. Can your partner control himself at work, at church, at the bank? Yes. Then he has the ability to control himself at home. Many who are abusive are referred to anger management programs. However, the problem is not the emotion of anger but the person's underlying beliefs.

The Power of Pornography

Pornography is an equal opportunity toxin. —Mary Anne Layden, PhD

It's no secret that men are visually aroused by women's bodies because they are trained early into that response, while women are less visually aroused and more emotionally responsive. The role of *pornography (porn)* in an abuser's life is huge because the industry is abusive (and society tolerates it).

"Pornography "comes from the New Testament word *porneia* which means "evil desire." The Hebrew word picture for "lust" *(ava)* means "the strong nail that hooks you to itself."

Porn makes the female body a site of dysfunction and assault. It teaches our boys that women are unworthy of respect, and valuable only as sex objects. There is a connection between porn and unwanted sexual coercion, violence, and rape. Studies state rapists act out the behavior they view;[155] and men who rape their partners usually view porn.[156]

Porn tells females that they must participate in painful sexual acts in order to keep a partner. Total control over another person is the power dynamic at the center of porn. Most porn movies, web sites, and magazines function as training manuals for abusers, whether they intend to or not.

It is also a fact that *the viewing of pornography is the seed that germinates the commercial sex industry.* The viewing of American movies and television seed and open the gateways to pornography. Pornography is said to be a Trojan horse sin, because it opens the door to other sexual sins. Today porn is not only a choice for adults but is being consumed in large numbers by our own children. Girls too are addicted to porn. Seventy-nine percent of youths' accidental and unsolicited exposure to porn occurs in the home.[157]

What we know is: In the world of porn, everything from the way people look to how and why they have sex is a *lie*. Remember, not all porn users will rape and abuse women. Those that do, rely on other values and beliefs to validate their actions.

To bring about change, the male attitude toward power and exploitation must be changed. It is therefore critical we teach our children that every person is made in the magnificent image of God. For our boys, we teach them to respect women and think critically about the culture's messages to which they're exposed.

An Abuser's Change Process

No doubt you have asked the second most common question, *"Can the abusive person I love change and become non-abusive?"* An abuser is often sincere in his promise to give up the use of abuse tactics—but, if the he/she has not relinquished their wish for power and control, the threat of abuse is still present. The guarantee of safety can never be based on a promise, no matter how heartfelt.

As much as our heart's desire may be for the abuser to change, it has been documented that it's exceedingly difficult for abusive people to alter their patterns of behavior. The recidivism rate for sexual abuse perpetrators is high. For many, remaining abusive is easier than stepping into a new pattern. Lundy Bancroft stated,

> If I were asked to select one characteristic of my abusive clients, an aspect of their nature that stands out above all others, I'd choose this one: They feel profoundly justified. Every effort to reach an abuser must be based on the antidote to this attitude. Abusers are *unwilling* to be non-abusive, not *unable*. They do not want to give up power and control. Counseling abusive men is difficult work. They are very reluctant to face up to the damage they've caused. They hold on tightly to their excuses and blame the victim. They become attached to various privileges they earn through mistreating their partners, and they have habits of mind that make it difficult to imagine being in a respectful and equal relationship with a woman.[158]

Often court-ordered treatment is done in groups, a setting where the offender is able to deny or minimize his actions; and able to fool others. On a rare occasion this person may promise to change, but he/she usually can't do it. On even rarer occasions, some work very hard and are able to change.

Sadly, most don't think they have a problem, so there will never be any change ... unless they ask Jesus into their life. One psychologist stated that more abusers are likely to participate in a comprehensive treatment program that does not label him as bad or sick or abusive.

Abusive behavior is like poison ivy, with its extensive deep root system. You can't eradicate it by lopping off the leaves. It must come out by the roots, which are the abuser's attitudes and beliefs regarding relationships. Since abuse is a learned behavior, the root causes of the deeply imbedded thoughts must be exposed and then unlearned; new behaviors must be learned. They, like all of us, need the powerful healing grace of God.

The real questions to be answered are, "Does he/she desire to change?" "Does he/she perceive their present behavior as abnormal?" And if they answer yes, "Will he/she actually do the work required?"

Intervention is often difficult because of the tendency for these people to think they don't have a problem, and therefore, drop out of treatment. Many abusers find more reasons to stay the same. The *benefits* far outweigh the pain of change: Power and control satisfy; he gets his way; he is the center of attention; receives free labor, sex, and freedom; enjoys victim status (casting themselves as abused abusers); financial control.[159] Is it any wonder they are reluctant to change?

To make genuine progress, the person needs to go through a critical set of steps that I call the *"Six R's to Authentic Change"*— *Recognizing, Rebuke, Responsibility, Remorse, Repentance,* and *Remaining.* See Appendix E.

Appendix E

THE SIX R'S TO AUTHENTIC CHANGE

> *For this people's heart has become calloused; they hardly hear with their ears, and they have closed their eyes. Otherwise they might see with their eyes, hear with their ears, understand with their hearts and turn, and I would heal them.*
> –Jesus, speaking in Matthew 13:15

> *"If we confess our sins, he is faithful and just and will forgive us our sins and purify us from all unrighteousness."* —John, speaking in 1 John 1:9

King David, a man after God's heart; a man who broke all the commandments, sinned horribly and felt the pain. He cried, *"The sacrifice you desire is a broken spirit. You will not reject a broken and repentant heart, O God"* (Psalm 51:17).

The key to significant change is facilitating a heart change, not simple behavior modification. To make genuine progress, the person needs to go through a critical set of steps that I call the *"Six R's to Authentic Change"*—*Recognizing, Rebuke, Responsibility, Remorse, Repentance,* and *Remaining.*

Recognize: For transformation to occur, the individual must recognize there's a problem, and express the desire or intent to change. They must see they're the ones creating their own problems in relationships; they are the ones holding onto distorted views—not others. This is followed by →

Rebuke. Successfully confronting the person who has harmed us and/or others involves a "rebuke" (means reprimand). Rebuke ought to *clarify the offense, its consequences, and the means for restoration.* He/she must listen to your perspective without interrupting, making excuses, or blaming his actions on you. They must admit what they did was wrong and sinful, a choice, and state they are willing to accept the consequences. This is followed by →

Responsibility: The person must be willing to take responsibility for their part, versus placing blame. Scripture says, *"Whoever lives by the truth comes into the light, so that it may be seen plainly that what they have done has been done in the sight of God"* (John 3:21). It is not wrong to expose a crime. It is more wrong to keep quiet. When a husband batters a wife, it is a crime. When a parent/caregiver abuses or neglects a child or senior in their care, it is a crime. When a pastor or a counselor becomes sexually involved with a counselee, it is a crime. Being a Christian doesn't exempt someone from being held legally accountable for their actions. Holding someone accountable is the most loving thing we could do. This is followed by →

Remorse: The definition of remorse is "feeling deep regret or guilt for a wrong committed." Remorse will often be accompanied by *deep and genuine* sadness, tears, apologies, promises to change, and possible self-punishment. The person needs to feel "broken" and begin the amends process. This is followed by →

Repentance: He/she must recognize that *all* have sinned and come short of the glory of God and need salvation and repentance (Romans 3:23). He/she must be more than remorseful. "Repentance" literally means to "change one's mind" or "to be converted." The person makes a 180-degree turn around and does the opposite of the problematic behavior. The repentant person agrees to make an *unconditional* agreement to immediately initiate behavior change (without you having to put pressure on him/her). For example, their lifestyle of lying is replaced with telling the truth in both big and small things.

Repentance takes time because deadly habits are difficult to unlearn and break. A habit, once strongly established, creates a brain map that reinforces itself and prevents other habits from being formed.[160] There will be successes, failures, and a lot of learning curves. Some will have periods of backwards movement or relapse. Relapse isn't failure, but a normal part of behavior change.

Change is always possible because humans can develop new brain maps that allow us to engage in godly behaviors, just as we engaged in sinful behaviors. And we can't overlook God's promise: *"I will give you a new heart, and I will put a new spirit in you. I will take out your stony, stubborn heart and give you a tender, responsive heart (Ezekiel 36:26).*

If the person is a believer, he/she is designed to be Christlike (means God manifested in and through us; our flesh). Going against a well-entrenched habit will be a challenge, but not impossible. God's Word encourages the person to keep on working until a Christlike brain is established.[161]

In his devotional *Daily Thoughts for Disciples,* Oswald Chambers stated that just because a person has altered his life (stopped being bad) that doesn't mean that he/she's truly repented. The repentant person is the one who becomes the opposite of what he/she was because Jesus Christ has put His own disposition into them, and it will be manifested in all he/she does. The disposition of Jesus can only enter a life by the way of repentance.[162]

Repentance is not:
- Measured by how much emotion the abuser shows or how many tears are shed.
- An abundance of gifts or good deeds.
- Arranged by someone else, such as a pastor or counselor; an act a church or court system requires.

Following repentance is the last "R." →
Remaining in recovery until the he/she is practicing the behavior successfully *and* there is the presence of truth. For example, if the person must show others that he/she habitually practices non-

addictive/abusive behavior for at least 6-months; one year is ideal; no lying, accusing or manipulating.

Even if the person is a believer, proper rehabilitation will likely be a lengthy, even a lifelong process. It can take several years to see appropriate results because it challenges underlying beliefs behind the behaviors. With abusers, professionals say that for life-long behavior changes to be realized, *the person must have practiced non-abusive behaviors for 5-years or more without relapse.*[163] As one psychologist put it, "Trust their behavior, not their words."

A changed heart and behaviors *over time* demonstrate repentance (Matthew 7:20; 1 Cor. 4:20). Casi wrote,

> *I'm so thankful my husband is changing. I know that doesn't happen very often. It's taken him years to rebuild my trust, but now I experience more peace and security. I've done the hard work too. I'm hopeful about our future. I pray our marriage will survive and grow stronger. But whatever happens, I know I will be okay.*

The God Who Loves

In a world without the law of God, you have chaos, oppression, and tyranny.
—Randy Terry, Operation Rescue

People who conceal their sins will not prosper, but if they confess and turn from them, they will receive mercy. –Proverbs 28:13

Does God love the Bill's and the predators of the world? This is a common question. Scripture clearly says God is love (1 John 4:8). God loves all people, but He doesn't always love what they do. There will always be consequences. (Read Psalm 15. The author warns of the consequences of using harsh abusive behaviors, while highlighting the benefits of healthy behaviors.)

Every person is lost. As Christians, we have the confidence that Jesus Christ can save and transform anybody. But you say, "[*Abuser name*] feels no conviction over his sin, is disrespectful, and dishonorable. When I talk to [*abuser*] about the issues he doesn't think he did anything wrong. He's totally unresponsive to me."

We may think this is an impossible situation to turn around, but Jesus doesn't. In the New Testament, we meet Zacchaeus. He was a "chief" tax collector. Tax collectors were despised by the public because they were Jews who were working for the hated Romans. They were viewed as traitors to their own countrymen. And they cheated the people they collected from. They would collect more than required and keep the extra for themselves. Luke 19:5-10 records Zacchaeus's encounter with Jesus,

> *Jesus looked up and said to him, "Zacchaeus, come down immediately. I must stay at your house today." So, he came down at once and welcomed him gladly. All the people saw this and began to mutter, "He has gone to be the guest of a sinner." But Zacchaeus stood up and said to the Lord, "Look, Lord! Here and now I give half of my possessions to the poor, and if I have cheated anybody out of anything, I will pay back four times the amount." Jesus said to him, "Today salvation has come to this house, because this man, too, is a son of Abraham. For the Son of Man came to seek and to save the lost."*

Who had been talking to Zacchaeus about his wrongdoings? No one. Did Jesus say anything about his corruption? No. What made him suddenly change and repent? The presence of Jesus. Jesus's desire is, "… *not wanting anyone to perish, but everyone to come to repentance" (2 Peter 3:9).*

Recognize that God loves *everyone*. Everyone deserves to be treated ethically and with respect—but *no one should be victimized*. Abusive people are human beings created in Gods' image who ended up on the wrong path.

"Repentance" and "to repent" are important biblical terms. Don't be put off by this "churchy" word. It simply means to *change one's attitudes and ways; to come to a right understanding*—as opposed to a wrong one. True biblical *repentance* is knowing what we did (past tense) was wrong; feeling a deep sorrow for sin, mixed with the resolve to begin writing a new healthy chapter of life.

Acts 3:19 reads, *"Repent, then, and turn to God, so that your sins may be wiped out, that times of refreshing may come from the Lord."* Repentance is a chance to start a fresh and headed in the right direction—in God's direction. The question is not whether the abuser can change, but does he/she *desire* to be transformed?

According to Dr. Stout, those with an *antisocial personality disorder* are often content with themselves and their lives and reject treatment. If they enter therapy, it's often because they have been court-referred, or there is a gain for them. Wanting to truly change is seldom the true reason they enter therapy.[164]

To make genuine progress, the person needs to go through a complex and critical set of steps that I call the *"Six R's to Authentic Change"*—*Recognizing, Rebuke, Responsibility, Remorse, Repentance,* and *Remaining,* which is outlined in Appendix E.

There's always hope, but *the desire to change is a must*. Meanwhile, we should pray for their souls. How does this make you feel?

MORE INFORMATION

If you want to connect with Kimberly, you can through her website at *www.OliveBranchOutreach.com* or on *Facebook*. Or, email her at *kim@kim-davidson.com*. If you are interested in learning more on abuse, there are additional topics covered on Kimberly's website: *OliveBranchOutreach.com*. Click on "Abuse Recovery" (on the left side) at *OliveBranchOutreach.com*.

ABOUT KIMBERLY

Kimberly Davidson lived two decades of her life in complete turmoil; in pain and addiction. Jesus heard the cry of her heart. He saw her pain and interceded, freeing her in 1989 from her personal prison. Today she calls herself a "wounded healer." She uses her voice, life wisdom from doing her own work, and pen to write curriculum and books for women in pain.

Kimberly is a board-certified biblical counselor, helping women mend their souls. She received her MA in specialized ministry from Western Seminary, Portland, Oregon; a BA in health sciences from the University of Iowa. She considers herself a lifelong learner. Kimberly has ministered to women for over 15-years, from within prison walls to youth centers, inspiring others to empower God to meet their emotional and spiritual needs.

She created *Olive Branch Outreach,* an interactive website dedicated to bring hope and restoration to those struggling with body image, abuse and food addiction. In addition, Kimberly leads an abuse recovery program at a federal women's prison. She is a consultant of abuse education for *Freedom Calling,* an anti-sex trafficking a ministry, and is a regular contributor to *Living in Truth,* a ministry that helps women who struggle with unhealthy eating and body image.

Kimberly lives in Oregon on a small ranch with her husband and critters.

BOOKS BY KIMBERLY

Every Body Remembers
Learn How to Get Past Your Past

No One Sent A Sympathy Card
The Grief that Goes Unrecognized
(A Biblical Response for Moving Beyond Life's Losses)

Turn Your Mind and Brain Back On
Unleash the Power of a Renewed Mind

I'm Beautiful? Why Can't I See It? [2nd Edition]
Love Yourself and Love Your Body in 12 Weeks

> **Eyes Wide Open**
> *Love Yourself and Love Your Body in 9 Weeks*
> (This is a shorter version of *I'm Beautiful? Why Can't I See It?*)

The Perfect Counselor
Break Through Your Past to Ensure a Healthy Future

I'm God's Girl? Why Can't I Feel It?
Daily Biblical Encouragement to Defeat Depression & the Blues

Something Happened On My Way to Hell
Break Free from the Insatiable Pursuit of Pleasure

Breaking the Cover Girl Mask: *Toss Out Toxic Thoughts*

Deadly Love: *Confronting the Sex Trafficking of Our Children*

Foundations *(A Parent's and Youth Leader's Guide)*
Empowering Youth to Establish Healthy Sexuality & Relationships

Torn Between Two Masters
Encouraging Teens to Live Authentically in a Celebrity-Obsessed World

My Notes

My Notes

References

[1] See: https://ncadv.org/statistics.
[2] Gavin DeBecker, *The Gift of Fear* (Little, Brown and Company, 1997) 8.
[3] *New York Times* 2011 report.
[4] Ibid, 9.
[5] Sociologist David Finkelhor conducted a massive study on child sexual abuse; http://www.indiaparenting.com/raising-children/
[6] https://online.rutgers.edu/awareness-of-domestic-violence-and-abusive-relationships/
[7] Mary Aiken, PhD, *The Cyber Effect* (New York: Spiegel & Grau, 2017), 211.
[8] Penny R. Smith, *The Second Woman Study* (Bloomington: WestBow, 2015) 111.
[9] Diane Langberg, *Christian Counseling Today*, "Shattered Innocence," Vol. 23 No 1, p. 20.
[10] Daniel Sweeny, Ph. D, *Traumatic Grief, Loss & Crisis 2.0*, "The Neurobiology of Childhood," Light University, 2015.
[11] Joe Navarro, *Dangerous Personalities* (New York: Rodale, 2014), 150.
[12] Alison Gopnik, *The Philosophical Baby*.
[13] EF Loftus, S. Polonsky & MT Fullilove, "Memories of Childhood Sexual Abuse," *Psychology of Women Quarterly* 18 no. 1, 1994.
[14] M.H. Silbet & A.M. Pines, "Early sexual exploitation as an influence in prostitution," *Social Work* (1983); 285-89; C.S. Wisdom & J.B. Kuhns, "Childhood victimization and subsequent risk for promiscuity, prostitution, and teenage pregnancy," *American Journal of Public Health,* 86 (1996): 1607-12.
[15] K.A. Tyler et al., "The impact of childhood sexual abuse on later sexual victimization among runaway youth," *Journal of Research on Adolescence,* 11 (2001): 151-76.
[16] https://www.disabilityscoop.com/2013/09/04/survey-abuse-widespread/18652/.
[17] Mike Lew, *Victims No Longer* (New York: Harper, 2004), 43.
[18] Matthew Lieberman, *Social: Why Our Brains Are Wired to Connect,* xi.
[19] Simon Baron-Cohen, *The Science of Evil* (New York: Basic Books, 2011) 6-11.
[20] Ibid, 6-20.
[21] Arlene Drake, *Carefontation* (New York: Regan Arts., 2017).
[22] Sometimes the God of the Old Testament (OT) doesn't sound like Jesus of the New Testament (NT). Jesus told His disciples, *"Who has seen me has seen the Father" (John 14:9).* When they looked into Jesus's face, they saw the essence of God. John's gospel states, "God is like Jesus." In other words,

God and Jesus are one. The God of the OT worked through the person of Jesus Christ in the NT. Let's not forget the Holy Spirit—the third person of the Trinity. Jesus said the Holy Spirit, our Helper and Counselor, would guide us into all truth (John 16:3). As God, the Holy Spirit truly functions as our Comforter and Counselor that Jesus promised He would be (John 14:16, 26, 15:26).

[23] Paraphrase from an anonymous email forward chain.

[24] W.D. Edwards, M.D., W.J. Gabel, M.Div., & F.E. Hosmer, M.S., "On the Physical Death of Jesus Christ," in JAMA: *The Journal of the American Medical Association,* 255, no. 11 (Mar 21, 1986), pp. 1457-58.

[25] Charles R. Swindoll, *The Darkness and the Dawn,* Insight for Living, 1982, p 62.

[26] Gavin DeBecker, *The Gift of Fear* (Little, Brown and Company, 1997) 108.

[27] Ibid, 26.

[28] Arlene Drake, *Carefontation* (New York: Regan Arts., 2017), 24.

[29] A. Newberg, MD & M. R. Walman, *How God Changes Your Brain* (New York: Ballantine Books, 2010), 141.

[30] Lundy Bancroft, *Why Does He Do That?* (New York: Berkley Books, 2002), 59.

[31] Gavin DeBecker, *The Gift of Fear* (Little, Brown and Company, 1997) 94-95.

[32] Deut. 22:25-26; Ezekiel 22:11, 13, 21; Lamentations 5:11, 21-22.

[33] Ibid.

[34] Joseph Hallinan, *Kidding Ourselves* (New York: Crown Publishers, 2014), 193.

[35] Gavin DeBecker, *The Gift of Fear* (Little, Brown and Company, 1997) 116.

[36] Matt Bays, *Finding God in the Ruins* (Colorado Springs: David C Cook, 2016), 124.

[37] *Child abuse* is when a parent or caregiver:

- Whether through action, or neglect or abandonment (mental illness, addiction, divorce), or commercial or other exploitation, causes injury, emotional harm, death, or risks serious harm to a child.
- Uses a too-harsh standard to judge by.
- Uses their position of power to take advantage of the child and gratify their own needs for importance, power, control, emotional and/or sexual gratification.

- Fight physically or verbally in front of the child. This is emotional abuse.

[38] DePrince et al., 2012.
[39] K. Kendall-Tackett; L. M. Ruglass, *Psycology of Trauma 101* (Springer, 2015), Chapter 9.
[40] Magnee MJ, Stekelenburg, JJ, Kemer C, de Gelder B, "Similar facial electromyographic responses …" *Neuroreport,* 2007, March 5; 18(4):369-72.
[41] Neuroscientists have discovered "mirror-neurons" in the brain that stimulate us unconsciously to imitate what we see; "Neurobiology of Imitation," 661-65.
[42] Strauss, Gelles, Steinmetz, *Behind Closed Doors* (New York: Anchor Books, 1980).
[43] Judith Herman, *Trauma and Recovery* (New York: Basic Books, 1997; 2015) 113.
[44] Sam Serio, *Sensitive Preaching to the Sexually Hurt* (Grand Rapids: Kregel, 2016) 108.
[45] Egeland, Jacobvitz & Sroufe, 1988.
[46] http://www.aish.com/jl/l/b/48966261.html
[47] Tim Harlow, *What Made Jesus Mad* (Nashville: Nelson Books, 2019), 109-111.
[48] Linda Graham, *Bouncing Back* (New World Library, 2013), xxv.
[49] Francine Shapiro, *Getting Past Your Past* (NY: Rodale, 2012), 14.
[50] Sandra L. Brown, *Counseling Victims of Violence* (Alexandria: American Association for Counseling and Development), 1991), 9.
[51] Aviva Romm, MD, *Adrenal Thyroid Revolution* (HarperOne Publishers, 2017) 54.
[52] Patrick J. Carnes, *Betrayal Bonds* (Deerfield Beach: Health Comm., 1997), 26.
[53] V.S. Ramachandran, *Phantoms in the Brain: Probing the Mysteries of the Human Mind.*
[54] Judith Herman, M. D., *Trauma and Recovery* (New York: Basic Books, 1997; 2015), 109.
[55] Stated on www.AddictionInfo.org: See http://www.addictioninfo.org/articles/4198/1/Is-Everyone-Addicted-To-Something/Page1.html; Accessed March 13, 2012.
[56] The basic working unit of the nervous system is a cell called a *neuron* or nerve cell. The human brain contains about 100 billion neurons. Think of it this way: We're all connected by the Internet, just like neurons in our brains. A neuron consists of a cell body containing the *nucleus,* and special extensions called *axons* and *dendrites* that receive and transmits signals.

A *synapse* is a structure that permits a neuron to pass an electrical or chemical signal to another neuron.

[57] Ai AL, Peterson C, Tice TN, H.B. Rodgers, Bolling SF: The influence of prayer coping on mental health among cardiac patients; J Health Psychol. 2007 Jul; 12(4), 580-96.

[58] Caroline Leaf, "How Prayer Affects the Brain: Prayer & Healing."

[59] Stated by Drs. Timothy Jennings and Caroline Leaf.

[60] Charles Duhigg, *The Power of Habit*.

[61] James Pennebaker, University Texas, *Opening Up By Writing It Down*.

[62] Stacey Colino, Health.USNews.com; August 31, 2016.

[63] Brian F. Martin, *Invincible* (New York: Perigee, 2014), 33, 45.

[64] Brene Brown, *Daring Greatly* (NY: Gotham Books, 2012) 45-46.

[65] Louann Brizendine, M.D, *The Female Brain,* (Broadway Publishing, 2007), 70-71

[66] "Image of God" is my addition; Linda Graham, *Bouncing Back* (Novato: New World Library, 2013), 284.

[67] N.I. Eisenberger and M.D. Lieberman, "Why rejection hurts," 294-300, *Trends in Cognitive Science,* 2004: 8 (7):

[68] Joe S. McIlhaney, Jr., M.D. and Freda McKissic Bush, M.D., *Hooked*, (Chicago: Northfield Publishing, 2008), 62, 43

[69] Kathryn Spink, *Mother Teresa: A Complete Authorized Biography* (HarperOne, 2011), 86.

[70] Jasmin L Cori, *The Emotionally Absent Mother* (The Experiment, 2010; 2017) 15-18.

[71] David J. Wallin, *Attachment in Psychotherapy* (New York: Guilford Press, 2007), n. 1. P. 24.

[72] Marnie Ferree, "Women and Pornography Today," *Christian Counseling Today,* Vol. 22, No. 1, 2017, 50.

[73] Jasmin Lee Cori, *The Emotionally Absent Mother* (New York: The Experiment, 2010; 2017) 46; 48.

[74] Louann Brizendine, *The Female Brain* (New York: Broadway Books, 2006), 19-20.

[75] Sue Gerhardt, *Why Love Matters,* 65-79.

[76] Robin Karr-Morse work; Donna Jackson Nakazawa, *Childhood Disrupted* (NEW YORK: Atria, 2105), 123.

[77] Regina Robertson, Editor, *He Never Came Home* (Chicago: Bolden, 2017), 23-26.

[78] Ibid, 28-29.

[79] Mary Aiken, PhD, *The Cyber Effect* (New York: Spiegel & Grau, 2017), 90-99.

[80] N.I. Eisenberger and M.D. Lieberman, "Why rejection hurts," 294-300, *Trends in Cognitive Science,* 2004: 8 (7):

[81] Louann Brizendine, *The Female Brain* (NY: Broadway Books, 2006), 67, 75-6.
[82] *Science*, October 10th issue, http://mentalhealth.about.com/b/2003/10/16/rejection-feels-like-pain-to-the-brain.htm
[83] Anne Moir, *Brain Sex: The Real Difference Between Men and Women,* 33-37, New York: Dell Publishing, 1991
[84] Paula Rinehart, *Sex and the Soul of a Woman* (Grand Rapids: Zondervan, 2010), 33.
[85] Joseph Hallinan, *Kidding Ourselves* (New York: Crown Publishers, 2014), 91.
[86] Don Hennessey, *How He Gets Into Her Head* (Cork, Ireland: Atrium, 2012), 18-22.
[87] Bob Sorge, *Dealing with the Rejection and Praise of Man,* "Rejection: God's Specialty" (Greenwood: Oasis House, 2002) 24.
[88] Alan D. Wolfelt, *The PTSD Solution* (Fort Collins: Companion Press, 2015) 20-21.
[89] Ibid.
[90] George A. Bonanno, *The Other Side of Sadness* (New York: Basic Books, 2009) 58.
[91] Linda Graham, *Bouncing Back* (New World Library, 2013), 263.
[92] Katherine Wollard, *Body/Mind,* "Go Ahead, Cry Yourself a River," from William Frey II, *Crying: The Mystery of Tears*
[93] Valerie E. Whiffen, *A Secret Sadness,* 39, Oakland: New Harbor Publications, 2006
[94] Dave Pelzer, *A Child Called It,* (Deerfield Beach, Health Communications, 1993), 139-140.
[95] Bob Sorge, *Dealing with the Rejection and Praise of Man,* "Your Source of Acceptance" (Greenwood: Oasis House, 2002).
[96] Ibid, p. 40
[97] Ibid, 85.
[98] Joe Navarro, *What Every Body is Saying* (New York: HarperCollins, 2008) 29, 206-207.
[99] Michelle Stevens, *Scared Selfless* (New York: G.P. Putnam's Sons, 2017) 6-7, 17.
[100] Sam Serio, *Sensitive Preaching to the Sexually Hurt* (Grand Rapids: Kregel, 2016) 33.
[101] Dr. Henry Cloud, Changes That Heal (Grand Rapids: Zondervan 1992) 121.
[102] Paula Rinehart, *Sex and the Soul of a Woman* (Grand Rapids: Zondervan, 2010), 36.

[103] Lisa Bevere, *Kissed the Girls and Made Them Cry* (Nashville: Nelson, 2002), 122.

[104] See: http://www.flurtmag.com/2013/08/a-culture-saturated-in-sex; 2013.

[105] Stephen R. Tracy & Celestia G. Tracy, *Princess Found,* Mending the Soul, 2011, 8.

[106] Douglas Brinkley, Rosa Parks: A Life (New York: A Penguin Life, 2000), 15.

[107] Bond & DePaulo, *Personality and Social Psychology Review,* Accuracy of deception judgments (2006), pp. 214-34.

[108] Fredrike Bannink, *Post Traumatic Success* (W.W. Norton & Company, 2014) 174.

[109] See: http://www.nytimes.com/2012/03/24/your-money/why-people-remember-negative-events-more-than-positive-ones.html?_r=0

[110] Caroline Leaf, *Who Switched Off My Brain,* (Switch On Your Brain; 2007), 8, 113-114, 94.

[111] Newberg and Waldman, *How God Changes Your Brain,* 39.

[112] Source: Dr. Caroline Leaf; TBN, May 25, 2016

[113] Gillath, Shaver, Wendleken, Mikulincer, "Attachment-style differences in the ability to suppress negative thoughts," *Neurimage.* 2005 Dec; 28 (4): 835-47

[114] www.westernseminary.edu/files/publications/magazine/WS_Magazine_Fall2016.pdf.

[115] Linda Graham, *Bouncing Back* (New World Library, 2013), 11-13.

[116] Source: Dr. Caroline Leaf; TBN, "The Disordered Mind;" March 9, 2016.

[117] See Leviticus 19:18; Deuteronomy 32:35; Proverbs 15:3. 24:12; Jeremiah 17:10; Nahum 1:3; Romans 12:17-21; 1 Thessalonians 5:15; Hebrews 10:30.

[118] Joseph Hallinan, *Kidding Ourselves* (New York: Crown Publishers, 2014), 88-89.

[119] Seth Gillihan, *Cognitive Behavioral Therapy Made Simple* (Althea Press, 2018), 75.

[120] Norman Doidge, "On Neuroplasticity."

[121] Lisa M. Najavits, *Seeking Safety* (The Guilford Press, 2002), 289.

[122] John M. Gottman, *The Seven Principles for Making Marriage Work.*

[123] Louann Brizendine, *The Female Brain* (New York: Broadway Books, 2006), 128.

[124] Goleman, 1995; 207.

[125] Tim Clinton & Mark Laaser, *The Fight for Your Life,* (Destiny Image, 2015), 60.

[126] L.R. Squire and E.R. Kandel, *Memory From Mind to Molecules* (New York: Scientific American Library, 2000).

[127] Peter A. Levine, *Trauma and Memory,* (Berkley: North Atlantic Books, 2015), 135.
[128] David Stoop, *You Are What You Think* (Spire Books, 1996), 58.
[129] Milan & Kay Yerkovich, *How We Love Our Kids* (Colorado Springs: WaterBrook Press, 2011), 281.
[130] Patrick Carnes, *Betrayal Bonds* (Deerfield Beach: Health Comm., 1997), 199-200.
[131] See: http://y98.cbslocal.com/2016/07/14/why-we-lie-about-our-relationship-status-on-social-media/
[132] William Glasser, *Choice Theory: A New Psychology of Personal Freedom* (1998), 35.
[133] Ibid. 24-28.
[134] See: http://dictionary.reference.com/browse/oppression?s=t.
[135] See: John 4:25-26; 11:1-44; 12:1-8; 20:1-16; Matt. 27:55-56; 27:61; Acts 1:14; 5:14; 8:12; 17:4, 12; 16:13-15; 1 Cor. 16:19.
[136] Henry Cloud & John Townsend, *Boundaries,* (Grand Rapids: Zondervan, 1992).
[137] Bill Eddy, *5 Types of People Who Can Ruin Your Life,* (Tarcher Perigee Book, 2018), 46.
[138] Martha Stout, *The Sociopath Next Door* (NY: Harmony Books, 2005), 109, 160.
[139] Stated by Lundy Bancroft; J. Cory & K. McAndless-Davis, *When Love Hurts* (New York: New American Library, 2016), xv.
[140] Joe Navarro, *What Every Body is Saying* (New York: HarperCollins, 2008) 67.
[141] Mary Aiken, PhD, *The Cyber Effect* (New York: Spiegel & Grau, 2017), 288.
[142] Ibid, 197.
[143] Joe Navarro, *Dangerous Personalities* (New York: Rodale, 2014), 187.
[144] Quoted by Joe Navarro, *Dangerous Personalities* (New York: Rodale, 2014), 64.
[145] Lundy Bancroft, *Why Does He Do That?* (New York: Berkley Books, 2002), 8, 70.
[146] Ibid, 9.
[147] John Cloud, "Minds on the Edge," *Time* (January 19, 2009), 42-46.
[148] Lundy Bancroft, *Why Does He Do That?* (NY: Berkley Books, 2002), 41-42.
[149] Ibid, 67.
[150] Ibid.
[151] Bill Eddy, *5 Types of People Who Can Ruin Your Life* (Tarcher Perigee Book, 2018) 19-20.
[152] Ibid, 33.
[153] Oswald Chambers, "Daily Thoughts for Disciples."

[154] Lundy Bancroft, *Why Does He Do That?* (New York: Berkley Books, 2002), 191, 200-203.
[155] Sam Serio, *Sensitive Preaching to the Sexually Hurt* (Grand Rapids: Kregel, 2016), 130.
[156] Ibid, 88.
[157] T. Clinton & M. Laaser, *The Fight of Your Life,* (Shippensburg: Destiny Image, 2014) 32.
[158] Lundy Bancroft, *Why Does He Do That?* (New York: Berkley Books, 2002), 376, xvii, 75.
[159] Ibid, 152-156.
[160] Norman Doidge, *The Brain that Changes Itself,* (New York: Penguin Books, 2007), 114-115.
[161] Michael Ginnis, *Signature Sins,* (IVP Books, 2011).
[162] Oswald Chambers, *Daily Thoughts for Disciples,* March 21, (Oswald Chambers Publications, 1994).
[163] According to the *Transtheoretical Model of Change (TTM)* developed by Dr. James Prochaska.
[164] Martha Stout, *The Sociopath Next Door* (NY: Harmony Books, 2005), 12-13.

Made in the USA
Columbia, SC
28 August 2019